HIV/AIDS Treatment in Resource Poor Countries

Yichen Lu · Max Essex · Chris Chanyasulkit
Editors

HIV/AIDS Treatment
in Resource Poor Countries

Public Health Challenges

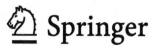 Springer

Editors
Yichen Lu
Department of Immunology
 and Infectious Diseases
Harvard School of Public Health
Boston, MA, USA

Max Essex
Department of Immunology
 and Infectious Diseases
Harvard School of Public Health
Boston, MA, USA

Chris Chanyasulkit
Department of Immunology
 and Infectious Diseases
Harvard School of Public Health
Boston, MA, USA

ISBN 978-1-4899-8581-1   ISBN 978-1-4614-4520-3 (eBook)
DOI 10.1007/978-1-4614-4520-3
Springer New York Heidelberg Dordrecht London

Printed on acid-free paper

Springer is part of Springer Science+Business Media (www.springer.com)

Foreword

December 1, 2011, was the 24th annual World AIDS Day. This one was particularly significant as 2011 marked the 30th anniversary of the first diagnosis of an AIDS patient. The organizers of World AIDS Day launched a 5-year campaign entitled "Getting to Zero," a theme that was meant to encompass the goals of zero new HIV infection, zero discrimination, and zero AIDS-related deaths.

Many high-profile people, politicians in particular, chimed in to echo the ambitious goals of the campaign. Hilary Rodham Clinton said that an AIDS-free generation was finally achievable. President Obama declared "we can beat this disease" and spoke of "the beginning of the end" of AIDS. Carla Bruni-Sarkozy spoke of her "dream of an HIV-free generation in the next few years—and of all generations being HIV-free from then on."

No politician ever wants to be a wet blanket. Yet behind their upbeat rhetoric, a sense of realism hangs in the air. Absent from the cacophony of celebratory remarks was a single confident voice asserting that there is a scientifically credible, or even plausible case that 30 years on, the end of the war against AIDS was in sight. The multitude of articles and commentaries in the press shared the tone of a writer putting on a brave face, putting aside his trepidation and exercising restraint in his language.

As usual, the politicians' words were neither all true nor all false. Whether the anti-HIV/AIDS enterprise has been a success or a failure depends on how one looks at it—from the viewpoint of curative medicine or from the viewpoint of public health.

As far as medicine goes, indeed, great progress has been made. Dispelling the ignorance and therefore the mystery and fear surrounding the cause of the disease 30 years ago, the viral etiology was established and the virus was isolated. This made it possible for the HIV infection to be diagnosed long before a patient enters into the phase of full-blown AIDS. With the availability of antiretroviral drugs, life expectancy from diagnosis of infection can now be measured in decades. During much of that time, a patient's viral load can be suppressed, the decline of CD4 cells can be reversed, and the onset of full-blown AIDS can be pushed back. For a patient who has access to good medical care, HIV infection can be regarded as a chronic disease which can be managed for years by medication even though the virus, integrated into the genome of certain host cells, is never entirely purged from the patient's body. The clinical course of an HIV-infected patient today can be worlds apart from that in the early days of AIDS. The strides made in understanding the biology of the virus and the mechanism of its pathogenesis, and in developing tools to diagnose and treat an HIV infection, comprise one of the most brilliant chapters in the annals of modern medicine.

The success in treating HIV patients came through the development of new drugs. Nucleoside analogs had already been developed in the 1970s for treating Herpes virus infection and cancer. Following in this pathway, new nucleoside analogs were developed to inhibit the replication of the HIV virus. Later, novel drug development techniques such as structural biology and computational chemistry were used to develop small molecule protease inhibitors and nonnucleoside reverse transcriptase inhibitors. Biologics were also developed such as peptides which inhibit viral entry into the host cell. The concerted efforts in developing anti-HIV drugs, targeting different parts of the virus' life cycle, have resulted in over 20 antiretroviral drugs approved by the FDA for treating HIV infection. Just as new drugs were discovered to treat one disease after another in the history of medicine, effective and safe drugs were successfully developed to treat HIV infection.

Whereas the practice of medicine addresses the health status of an individual patient, the practice of public health addresses the disease burden on a whole population. Central to the mission of public health is the control of the spread of HIV infection such that the pandemic can be extinguished. The major concerns are the incidence and prevalence of diseases, the systems for provisioning healthcare, and the economics thereof. In contrast to the great strides made in treating a patient infected with HIV, the public health scorecard in dealing with the HIV/AIDS problem is mixed. The greatest success was achieved in stopping mother-to-child transmission of the virus where zero infection does look to be achievable. The broader picture, however, is less encouraging. As of 2010, there were still 2.7 million people around the world who became newly infected with HIV, adding to a prevalence of 33 million people worldwide who were already living with HIV infection. Of these, only 6.6 million were getting treatment. Regional differences in prevalence also paint a grave picture. In three southern African countries, the prevalence of HIV infection in the adult population exceeds 20%.

Traditional public health measures used to deal with pandemics have been much less usable in dealing with the HIV pandemic. Quarantine, probably the most effective public health measure used to extinguish pandemics beside vaccination, did not work in the case of HIV because infections remain asymptomatic and often unknown for years after exposure. A good contrast is between HIV and SARS. SARS is a disease with rapid symptomatic manifestations after infection. Upon the discovery of the emergence of a new infectious disease, the world immediately mounted a quarantine response which stopped the spread of the disease. With HIV infection, this was not possible. It is estimated that in the USA, 20% of the infected do not even know that they are infected and they carry on activities which infect others. In sub-Saharan Africa, that percentage is sure to be higher.

Viewing from these two different vantage points, the track record of the HIV/AIDS enterprise can indeed be classified both as a success and a failure—a success by the standard of medicine, a failure by the standard of public health. This is not to say that progress has not been made on the public health front, but the world is far from bringing the pandemic under control.

Theoretically, there is no reason why the success in curative medicine for HIV infection cannot be rolled out to become a public health success. Practically, what stands in the way is economics. The world now has the knowledge and the tools to stop the spread of the HIV virus, but not the means committed to do so.

In 2003, President George W. Bush initiated the President's Emergency Program for AIDS Relief (PEPFAR) which allocated 15 billion dollars to making antiretroviral drugs available in developing countries. In 2008, the US Congress passed an appropriation bill to authorize up to 48 billion dollars for the next 5 years to combat global HIV/AIDS, tuberculosis, and malaria. Together with the Global Fund to Fight AIDS, Tuberculosis and Malaria and private foundations such as the Gates Foundation and the Clinton Foundation, there are now about seven billion dollars each year available for treating HIV patients in low and middle income countries. The impact of this sum was further maximized by aggressive negotiation with pharmaceutical companies to lower the cost of antiretroviral drugs. The annual cost for each patient is now down to $335. Fifteen years ago, antiretroviral drugs cost $10,000 per annum. It is a great accomplishment that there are now 6.6 million people worldwide who have access to treatment for AIDS. Of that number, five million are in sub-Saharan Africa where only 20,000 were being treated in 2004. Impressive as this number is, it still pales in comparison with the estimate that 14.2 million AIDS patients worldwide are sick enough to be put on treatment.

A still more foreboding statistic is that for every person who is newly put on treatment now, there are two persons who are becoming newly infected with HIV. Since the use of antiretroviral drugs is lifelong and the median age of diagnosis of HIV infection is in the 20s or 30s depending on the country, even a conservative treatment protocol would mean that the addition of each newly infected person creates an additional financial burden for a decade or more of treatment some time down the road. The more the antiretroviral therapies prolong the lives of the HIV infected, the greater is the number of years of drug treatment needed for each patient. The financial burden for HIV treatment worldwide is therefore increasing exponentially. The sheer math is sobering. It is no wonder that a certain pessimism has set in that the war against AIDS cannot be won.

Ongoing clinical studies continue to come up with new ways of using the antiretroviral drugs for greater benefit. Most notable is the HPTN 052 clinical trial which was halted in May 2011 by the independent Data and Safety Monitoring Board for ethical reasons because the data were so overwhelming that initiating HIV-positive patients on antiretroviral therapy when their CD4 counts were in the 350–500 cells/μL range as opposed to waiting until their CD4 counts declined to 250 cells/μL had an effect of reducing by 96% the risk of transmission of the virus to the HIV-uninfected partners of the HIV-serodiscordant couples in the trial. The benefit to the health status of the HIV positive partner of these couples seen in this trial strengthens emerging evidence that treating early is better than treating late. Now, imagine the financial ramification of putting HIV-positive patients on therapy earlier than what is being practiced now! Herein is another example of a medical breakthrough in the treatment of HIV patients which will have a problematic future as a public health measure at the population level for reason of sheer economics.

Given that there are not enough medicines to go around, the fair allocation of drugs becomes a question loaded with bioethical questions. Does making drugs available in one part of the world, or to one particular high-risk group, have greater impact in stopping the spread of HIV globally? What is the role of personal responsibility in risky behaviors which lead to acquisition of the infection or transmission of the infection to others? Who bears the responsibility for drug compliance for those who are under treatment? In countries with socialized medicine, how should resources be prioritized in the treatment of acute versus chronic diseases or one disease versus another? Policy considerations are fraught with conundrums and the choices are exceedingly difficult.

Government agencies remain the largest source of funding for HIV treatment. In democratic countries, the use of the country's financial resources is subject to the constraints of democratic institutions and processes and is hence subject to the collective political will of the populace. In the early days of the HIV pandemic, there was a sense of exigency in the western countries and therefore a groundswell of popular support for governments to devote resources to combatting AIDS. With the passage of time, that sense of exigency has waned. The success of the antiretroviral drugs in treating HIV patients has also created an illusion that the AIDS pandemic is now under control. Combatting AIDS no longer enjoys the priority in the national agenda as it once did, all the more in recent years as the governments in the developed world have all fallen into extreme financial stress. With its own healthcare system financially unsustainable, it is doubtful that America will be as generous when the PEPFAR program comes up for renewal in 2013. In light of the latest census data showing that 46.2 million Americans are living under the poverty line, the highest number in the 52 years that the Census Bureau has been collecting income data on the American people, it is also doubtful that American largess towards the developing world will be as plentiful in the future. Difficult economic times breed isolationism.

As a result of the world financial crisis that began in 2008, philanthropic donations for the AIDS cause have also waned. Some of the formerly active NGOs devoted to the AIDS cause are now in financial straits. It is hard to be optimistic that there will be a massive infusion of new funds to support HIV treatment.

Equally discouraging is the poor prospect of a universal prophylactic vaccine against HIV. Weakly effective vaccines as the ALVAC/AIDSVAX vaccine tested in the Thailand trial are no cause for optimism. Such vaccines can never be deployed in real-life situations for fear that they create an illusion of protection which in turn encourages risky behavior. Even though there is the possibility that a conserved epitope on the HIV-1 envelope protein gp120 may give rise to neutralizing antibodies, the availability of a vaccine is realistically nowhere in sight. The prophylactic use of neutralizing antibodies is also unrealistic.

If neither a vaccine nor the adequate resources to fund HIV treatment appear imminent, the fight to contain the spread of HIV will have to resort to more traditional public health measures which have had proven efficacy at controlling diseases or improving health at the population level. One should not forget that changing the public's attitude and behavior through public education succeeded in reducing cigarette smoking. Coupled with light-touch legislations, the antismoking campaign in America produced one of the all-time success stories in public health. In the prevention of HIV infection, public education in using condoms has borne fruit with certain high-risk groups, as has the public education for injection drug users not to share needles.

Several randomized controlled trials in Africa have shown that male circumcision is highly effective in reducing heterosexual HIV transmission. In three trials, the data were so overwhelming they were terminated early for ethical reasons. Unlike the use of condom or vaginal microbicide which has to be done at every sexual encounter, male circumcision is done once for a lifetime benefit. In this regard, it is like a vaccine. Programs in Botswana and Swaziland have shown that male circumcision is welcome by both men and their female partners. There do not appear to be insurmountable cultural barriers to the idea of male circumcision. Being a surgical procedure, it is necessary to organize the delivery of male circumcision in a more cost-effective fashion. There is no reason why this cannot be done.

In both Uganda and Zimbabwe, there is evidence that reduction in casual sex and in the number of sexual partners—behavioral changes brought about by public campaigns—has also contributed to reducing HIV transmission. The field experience for male circumcision and for the reduction of concurrent sexual partners strongly argues for public education as a highly effective strategy for reducing HIV transmission. Such public education programs, rather mundane and never able to garner the limelight as scientific or medical breakthroughs, are actually more effective at the population level. There must be redoubling of efforts in such behaviorally based public health strategies.

On the healthcare delivery side, one should not forget that community-based efforts played a large role in reducing HIV infection among sex workers in many countries. The use of community-based efforts both to promote prevention and drug compliance among those who are under treatment should be supported.

In light of a high likelihood of declining funds available for providing antiretroviral therapy to the developing world, drug treatment programs should be adjusted to get the greatest benefit out of available resources. The antiretroviral drugs have now been in use for so long in such a large patient population that they are proven to be safe. In one study conducted by British scientist in three African countries, it was found that routine laboratory testing of the patients, hitherto thought to be necessary for monitoring toxicity and side effects of the drugs, conferred no additional survival benefit 5 years out. This so-called Lab-Lite approach is one way of shifting the available finances from routine lab testing to buying more drugs and making drugs available to people living in remote areas where healthcare facilities are not equipped to do the laboratory testing. The provisioning of drug treatment can be done more economically without eroding the quality of care.

Apart from prevention and treatment, the disease surveillance function of the public health infrastructure must not be overlooked. This vigilance is particularly critical because HIV comes in several subtypes and is hypermutable. New evidence is emerging that the HIV-1B subtype of the virus, prevalent in North America and Europe, has very different properties than the HIV-1C subtype which is prevalent in South Africa, the latter being much more efficient in heterosexual transmission and is found in high titers for a prolonged period after the acute phase of infection. The ramification of this latter property for disease control is profound. The surveillance infrastructure of the public health system must be strengthened to pick up different behaviors of the viral subtypes at the population level as well as the potential emergence of variant forms of the virus.

Finally, we should not give up hope that science will be able to deliver medically based means for controlling the spread of HIV at a cost that the world can afford. Funding for studying the virology and immunology of HIV should continue. Expenditures designed for current outcome must be balanced with expenditures designed for future payoff. It may seem like a long shot, but in light of the unbearable economics of antiretroviral treatment-based prevention strategies, it is a risk that we cannot afford not to take. The success of antiretroviral therapy should not stifle the exploration for new treatment and prevention modalities, especially modalities that can be mass deployed economically. We may do well to acknowledge the limitations of current therapies and apply fresh thinking to the problem.

The current research funding environment in America is certainly less than friendly. In the face of a declining NIH budget, funding any one area of research is at the expense of funding other areas of research. Considering AIDS is not even in the top 15 causes of death in the general population of America, the case is biased towards funding research on diseases which afflict a much larger percentage of the American population. With the aging of the Baby Boomers, there is a powerful demographic force in favor of supporting the study of diseases of the aged such as cancer, cardiovascular diseases, and neurodegenerative diseases. Diseases whose incidences are increasing at alarming rates are also more likely to garner funding. Obesity, metabolic syndrome, and diabetes are prime examples. Considering obesity afflicts one-third of all Americans while about one million American live with HIV, it is futile to assert, as one article headline on AIDS Day last year stated that "Belt-tightening can't apply to AIDS."

Looking back, the AIDS pandemic came on the scene at precisely the moment that the world was most confident about its ability to eradicate infectious diseases. It was in 1979 that WHO certified smallpox as extinct, a mere 12 years after WHO launched an intensive program to eradicate the disease. As late as the early 1950s, there were 50 million new cases of smallpox each year worldwide. It was in the face of such triumphalism that AIDS burst on the scene. Upon the discovery of the HIV virus in 1981, Margaret Heckler, then Secretary of Health and Human Services, declared in 1984 that an HIV vaccine would be tested in 2 years. Such hubris turned out to be foolhardy.

Throughout human history, man had always coexisted with pathogenic micro-organisms. Such is the design of nature. It is a struggle for survival between the microbes and the human race. From time to time, the pathogens would have the upper hand and a swathe of humanity would be wiped out from the face of the earth such as the bubonic plague which killed a third of the European population in the fourteenth century, or the Spanish flu pandemic of 1918 which killed at least 50 million people worldwide. Less spectacular but more frequent outbreaks of chol-era, measles, smallpox, influenza, typhus, and tuberculosis would claim tens of thousands or even millions of lives in each episode. In all cases, the human race survived and a new equilibrium was re-established between man and the patho-genic microbe. Other than smallpox, there has not been another infectious disease that has been eradicated throughout human history. Science, together with history, does not support a case that AIDS will be extinguished from the face of the earth. More than likely, the end game will be an uneasy equilibrium between man and the HIV virus.

While science and science-based modern medicine have done so much to improve the human lot, we must not be lulled into the false belief that science is omnipotent. For the battle with HIV/AIDS, we would do well to push the frontier of science as if it has no limits, but work with other approaches concurrently as if future science will not be able to deliver a solution, at least not one that will come soon enough. Sound and robust public health endeavors in dealing with the HIV/AIDS problem have never been more important to the continuing well-being of the human race.

Newton, MA, USA   Gerald L. Chan, Sc.D.
Boston, MA, USA

Preface

AIDS: A Public Health Crisis Forcing Improvement of Public Health Systems Worldwide

> If you understand AIDS, you understand public health. There's almost no aspect of behavior, policy, basic science, statistics, epidemiology, nutritional interventions—everything—that does not touch HIV/AIDS.
>
> Max Essex (Harvard Public Health Review, November 2011)

For public health workers in developing countries, working on AIDS prevention and control requires a broad range of social skills and special knowledge not taught in public health schools. Many of us from public health schools have often been impressed by what local AIDS workers in Africa and Asia have accomplished in terms of providing help to AIDS patients in resource-poor regions. Publishing this book is part of our continuous effort to encourage the world to learn about how and what these AIDS workers in developing countries have done in the fight against the AIDS pandemic, in the hope that with such encouragement, more and more public health students and workers will devote their careers to AIDS prevention and treatment. We also hope that this book will provide a source of inspiration for more people to become interested in various international or local AIDS programs anywhere or everywhere in the world. Unlike other infectious diseases that come and go, such as SARS in 2003 and the H1N1 "Swine Flu" in 2009, AIDS came to stay. The challenges facing AIDS workers today will surely face many generations of AIDS workers in the years to come.

Being an AIDS worker in a developing country or a resource-poor region might mean raising funds to build a clinic, a school, a nursing home, or even a paved road connecting a village to the outside world; or being a social activist fighting to obtain funds for public health costs from local or national governments; or a clinician who may need to be able to deal with any kind of medical emergency as the only doctor or nurse in the entire village. Treating AIDS patients effectively requires the most advanced modern medical knowledge. The new antiretroviral drugs are based on very recent scientific discoveries and created by major investments of research and development. Tens of thousands of AIDS workers have successfully used these drugs in developing countries and resource-poor regions to save lives and prevent newborn babies from being infected by their infected mothers. As described in this book, these AIDS workers often accomplished their mission in "impossible" environments, working under extremely harsh living conditions in places with no existing public health infrastructure.

The idea of publishing this book was conceived when we conducted our annual AIDS medical training courses and research workshops in China. Many of us from public health schools sat together trying to figure out which new medical training topics in antiretroviral (ARV) treatment and which new research discoveries we should bring in to each group of trainees. We, as instructors in these courses, were also students ourselves, as we learned from our trainees and from each other. We soon realized that public health students back home or around the world, some of whom will hopefully become future AIDS workers, could benefit from reading the presentations of these workshops. We decided to include one chapter to describe the prevention of mother-to-infant transmission in some remote villages in China where modern prenatal medical care did not previously exist, and one chapter to describe how free ARV treatment was started and maintained in some poor villages that lacked very basic public health infrastructure or even paved roads connecting them to the outside world. We included one of the most popular presentations in the past training courses where the trainees learned how India dealt with ARV treatment because AIDS workers in China faced similar challenges. We specifically selected a presentation that described the ARV treatment programs in Africa, which were made possible by the US President's Emergency Plain for AIDS Relief (PEPFAR). In order to elicit more strategic thinking about the future of the global ARV treatment program and for public health students to get prepared for more challenges to come, we included a chapter by some of the researchers who first proposed the concept of ARV prophylaxis. We also included a chapter by a Chinese national public health official that addresses improving access to generic ARV drugs through international collaboration and specific WTO rules. We also included a presentation trying to answer one of the most frequently asked questions in these workshops: when will most AIDS patients in the world have access to effective treatment?

The past 30 years of the AIDS pandemic have resulted in tens of millions of deaths, mostly in developing countries. This global tragedy will unfortunately continue into the foreseeable future. AIDS workers around the world have no choice but to fight this dreadful disease with any and all tools they may have or acquire. An encouraging thought is that in trying to treat AIDS patients under very difficult conditions, such AIDS workers have, at the same time, improved public health infrastructure. In some developing countries and resource-poor regions, AIDS workers are actually creating basic public health infrastructures that had eluded many generations of public servants before them. And the newly created public health services, despite their simplicities and need for improvement, provide foundations and hope for future generations.

Boston, MA, USA   Yichen Lu
                                                                   Max Essex

Acknowledgements

The editors thank Dr. Lendsey Melton for his enormous help with the editing process. Thanks also are due to Stephen Heim and Christopher Helmuth for departmental support; Alexandra Lu and Peter Lu for editorial assistance; Mei Zheng and Fu Yang for translation assistance; and Khristine Queja and her team, including Kathryn Hiler, at Springer Publishing for providing critical support and encouragement to this project. The editors would like to thank all of the instructors and trainees in the past annual Harvard AIDS medical training courses and research workshops, especially Drs. Gui Xien, Sandra Burchett, Roger Shapiro, Marcus Altfeld, Zhao Qingxia, Yu Lan, Zhang Fujie, and Sun Yongtao. Finally, the editors would like to thank the collaborative authors for their dedication of time and effort to this publication.

In preparing this volume, as in its other work, the Harvard School of Public Health's China Project relies on a grant support from the Office of AIDS Research (OAR) of the National Institutes of Health (NIH) to the Harvard School of Public Health's AIDS Initiative (HAI).

Contents

Contributors

Qingling Chen, M.D. Yunnan AIDS Care Center, Kunming, Yunnan, China

Xiaoduan Cheng Wolong Health Center, Shangcai County, Henan Province, China

Max Essex Department of Immunology and Infectious Diseases, Harvard School of Public Health, Boston, MA, USA

Phyllis J. Kanki Department of Immunology and Infectious Diseases, Harvard School of Public Health, Boston, MA, USA

Yunfei Lao, M.P.H. Yunnan AIDS Care Center, Kunming, Yunnan, China

Yichen Lu Department of Immunology and Infectious Diseases, Harvard School of Public Health, Boston, MA, USA

Kathrine Meyers, Dr.P.H. Aaron Diamond AIDS Research Center, New York, NY, USA

Vladimir Novitsky Department of Immunology and Infectious Diseases, Harvard School of Public Health, Boston, MA, USA

Haoyu Qian, M.P.H. Aaron Diamond AIDS Research Center, New York, NY, USA

Yiming Shao, M.P.H. State Key Laboratory for Infectious Disease Prevention and Control, National Center for AIDS/STD Control and Prevention, Chinese Center for Disease Control and Prevention, Beijing, China

Srikanth P. Tripathy National AIDS Research Institute, Pune, Maharashtra, India

Sriram P. Tripathy Indian Council of Medical Research, Jagtapnagar, Wanawadi, Pune, India

Nzovu Ulenga Department of Immunology and Infectious Diseases, Harvard School of Public Health, Boston, MA, USA

Zengquan Zhou, M.D. Yunnan AIDS Care Center, Kunming, Yunnan, China

Yunnan AIDS Initiative, Kunming, China

Chapter 1
Prevention of HIV Infection in the Absence of a Vaccine

Max Essex and Vladimir Novitsky

Introduction

It has been about 30 years since AIDS was first recognized as a new disease [1–3]. Within a year or two after the initial recognition of the disease in homosexual men, what appeared to be the same disease—severe and irreversible immunosuppression—was also recognized in other groups: injection drug users [4], hemophiliacs [5], blood transfusion recipients [6], a few infants [7], and people in Africa [8]. Within 2–3 years after the initial recognition of AIDS as a disease, the cause was identified, a new human lentivirus that was initially called human T-cell lymphotropic virus III [9], or lymphadenopathy-associated virus [10].

At the time HIV was identified as the cause of AIDS, many in the public health community thought that a vaccine against AIDS could be rapidly developed. Effective vaccines had already been developed against a wide variety of viral diseases. Despite more than 25 years of research, we are still many years away from the availability of an efficacious HIV vaccine.

Most other approaches for preventing the spread of HIV among adults have had only modest success. These include the broad categories of education and behavior change, condoms, and vaginal microbicides that contain broad-spectrum ingredients rather than antiretroviral drugs (ARVs) [11]. The circumcision of males has been moderately effective, with estimates of about 60% protection usually cited [12]. Other sexually transmitted infections, especially Herpes, are associated with increased risk for infection with HIV [13]. Yet the successful treatment of genital Herpes with acyclovir did not decrease risk of transmission of HIV [14]. When considered together, interventions to prevent HIV infection have been disappointing, especially in sub-Saharan Africa where the epidemic is most severe.

M. Essex (✉) • V. Novitsky
Department of Immunology and Infectious Diseases, Harvard School of Public Health
AIDS Initiative, 651 Huntington Avenue, Boston, MA 02115-6017, USA
e-mail: messex@hsph.harvard.edu; vnovi@hsph.harvard.edu

Y. Lu et al. (eds.), *HIV/AIDS Treatment in Resource Poor Countries:*
Public Health Challenges, DOI 10.1007/978-1-4614-4520-3_1,
© Springer Science+Business Media New York 2013

Southern Africa and HIV-1C

It has been estimated that more than 70% of the world's HIV infections are in sub-Saharan Africa, which represents about 10% of the world population (Table 1.1a). Prevalence rates of HIV are particularly high in southern Africa, perhaps 3–5 times higher than the other regions of sub-Saharan Africa, where it has been estimated that up to 25% of adults aged 15–49 may be infected in some countries [15]. The southern African region has more than one-third of the world's HIV infections, with less than 2% of the world's population. The country of South Africa has about one-quarter of all infections in sub-Saharan Africa, with just 6% of the population in sub-Saharan Africa (Table 1.1b).

Table 1.1 Estimated prevalence of HIV in adults, 2009

(a) Geographical regions

Region	Population[a]	% of world population[a]	Mean prevalence[b]	Total infections[a]	% of world infections
World	6,792.89	100	0.8	33.3	100
Asia	3,771.39	55.5	0.1	4.9	14.6
Sub-Saharan Africa	788.23	11.6	5.0	22.5	67.6
Southern	134.37	2.0	13.9	11.3	33.9
East	133.38	2.0	5.6	4.5	13.5
West	298.83	4.4	2.7	4.7	14.1
Western and Central Europe	607.81	8.9	0.2	0.8	2.4
North America	451.71	6.6	0.5	1.5	4.5
Central and South America	431.42	6.4	0.5	1.4	4.2
Middle East and North Africa	292.92	4.3	0.2	0.5	1.4
Eastern Europe and Central Asia	273.20	4.0	0.8	1.4	4.2
Caribbean	35.23	0.5	1.0	0.2	0.7

(b) Estimated prevalence of HIV in adults, selected countries in sub-Saharan Africa, 2009

Country	Population[a]	% SSA population	Mean prevalence[b]	Total infections[a]	% SSA infections
Botswana	1.99	0.3	24.8	0.3	1.4
Burkina Faso	15.75	2.1	1.2	0.1	0.5
Kenya	39.71	5.2	6.3	1.5	6.7
Malawi	15.03	2.0	11.0	0.9	4.1
Nigeria	157.47	20.5	3.6	3.3	14.7
Senegal	12.01	1.6	0.9	0.1	0.3
South Africa	49.05	6.4	17.8	5.6	24.9
Swaziland	1.34	0.2	25.9	0.2	0.8
Tanzania	41.05	5.3	5.6	1.4	6.2
Uganda	32.37	4.2	6.5	1.2	5.3

[a]In millions
[b]In adults, from UNAIDS [15]

The reasons why the epidemic is so much more severe in southern Africa are not clear. They may include lower rates of male circumcision and different patterns of sexual behavior, such as multiple concurrent partnerships [16], but increasing evidence also suggests that HIV-1C, the viral subtype that dominates in the area, may be more transmissible by heterosexual contact [17]. The HIV-1C of southern Africa has extra NFkB sites in the long terminal repeat region of the virus, which enhance transcriptional activation [18]. The HIV-1C virus envelope maintains high affinity for infection through the CCR5 coreceptor on macrophage and T4 lymphocyte cell membranes [19]. By contrast, HIV-1B and HIV-1D, which seem less efficiently transmitted, often evolve to lose CCR5 tropism after prolonged periods of infection, to become dependent on the CXCR4 coreceptor. This may be particularly important for infection via the reproductive tract, where it appears that only CCR5-type viruses are infectious because cells with the other major co-receptor, CXCR4, are not present at the mucosal surfaces of the reproductive tract [20]. Langerhans cells, which probably represent the main target for infection at the vaginal junction with the uterine cervix, and in the foreskin of the penis, are easier to infect with CCR5-type viruses [21]. Higher overall viral loads (VLs) have also been reported for HIV-1C [22, 23], and this virus grows better in gut-associated lymphoid tissues, which are thought to be a primary site for initial expansion of the infection [24].

Treatment with Antiretroviral Drugs

In contrast with the lack of success in making an HIV vaccine, it was soon clear that ARVs could be used to treat people with HIV/AIDS. By about 1988, the first drug, zidovudine (ZDV), was available [25]. Within 5 or 6 years, various new drugs that acted on the viral reverse transcriptase or on the viral protease were available. It was soon clear that the drugs could save the lives of AIDS patients when used in appropriate combinations. All the drugs worked by blocking the intracellular replication of HIV, lowering VL so that little virus was left to kill immune cells. By 1994, it was also apparent that ZDV given to an HIV-positive pregnant woman could reduce the risk that she would infect her child during gestation or delivery [26], setting the precedent that such drugs could be used for prophylaxis.

Despite evidence that the drugs worked so well in the USA and Europe, they would not be widely available in most developing countries for many years. The drugs were expensive, and many international health experts were not convinced that they could be used effectively outside of modern hospital settings. There was concern that patients in developing countries might not be as adherent to the required schedules for taking pills, and lack of adherence was known to give rise to drug resistance. The HIVs in Africa were also different subtypes, and little was known about how the viral sequence differences might affect rates and patterns of drug-resistance development, as well as the fitness for transmission of drug-resistant variants.

Although some differences in drug-resistance patterns were observed with HIV-1C in southern Africa, it was soon apparent that the treatment of AIDS patients with ARVs could be just as effective in Africa as in the USA and Europe, assuming drugs were available [27]. By 2002 or 2003, many countries in Africa began using ARVs in limited populations. International governmental and nongovernmental donor organizations succeeded in obtaining deep reductions in drug prices, and the funding for programs to provide free drugs, such as the President's Emergency Plan for AIDS Relief (PEPFAR) and the Global Fund, became available. In Africa, about one-third of HIV-infected people who need drugs for clinical AIDS may be receiving these drugs. In some countries, such as Botswana and Namibia, a much larger proportion of AIDS patients receive the drugs. Typical criteria for initiation of highly active antiretroviral treatment (HAART) are an AIDS-defining illness and/ or a lowering of CD4 count to 200 or 250, though more countries are now considering initiation when CD4 levels fall below 350. Typical three-drug combinations used have been Trimmune—a formulation including stavudine (d4T), lamivudine (3TC), and efavirenz (EFV)—or combivir, which includes ZDV with 3TC, and either nevirapine (NVP) or EFV. More recently, the combinations of d4T and 3TC or ZDV and 3TC are increasingly replaced with Truvada, which is a two-drug combination of tenofovir and emtricitabine, as the latter combination may cause fewer early side effects.

Prevention of Mother-to-Child Transmission

Following the evidence that ZDV alone could reduce mother-to-child transmission (MTCT) when given in utero in the developed world [26], various approaches were tested for prevention of mother-to-child transmission (PMTCT) in developing country settings. These ranged from dosing with ZDV for longer vs. shorter periods in late gestation and immediately after birth in Thailand, to a trial in Uganda that tested whether NVP chemoprophylaxis could still reduce MTCT if given only when the mother first presented at the time of labor [28]. Surprisingly, even when NVP was only given at birth, it still reduced MTCT by up to 50%. This was thought to be particularly important for poor country settings where pregnant women often did not come to health clinics until very late in gestation.

Other studies showed that using more drugs worked better than using fewer drugs [29, 30], and that drugs given to breastfeeding infants could also lower the risk of infant infections that occurred through the mother's milk [30, 31]. In all cases, there was a strong correlation between reductions in viral RNA levels in blood and breast milk and reduced risk that the infant would be infected at any of the three stages of risk: gestation, delivery, and breastfeeding. The most dramatic reductions in MTCT occurred when the mother was initiated on three-drug HAART by week 27 of gestation and remained on HAART while breastfeeding [30]. Even though this resulted in very low levels of viral RNA in milk, it did not cause lower levels of cell-associated proviral DNA [32], and earlier studies suggested that some breastfeeding

MTCT might be due to cell-associated DNA [33]. Nonetheless, the results when HAART was used throughout breastfeeding and the last one-third of gestation were dramatic, with less than 1% of infants becoming infected with at least two different three-drug HAART regimens [30]. These reductions were as great as those seen with chemoprophylaxis used during pregnancy in developed countries, even when formula was used in place of breastfeeding. Formula feeding to replace breastfeeding was also tested in some developing countries, but usually abandoned because the use of unclean water to prepare the formula resulted in unacceptable rates of other water-borne diseases [31].

Antiretroviral Drugs to Prevent Sexual Transmission

With the recognition that most prevention interventions that did not include ARVs were insufficiently effective, and that ARVs worked very well in developing countries for both AIDS treatment and PMTCT, enthusiasm also rose for using ARVs for prevention of adult infections. Potential interventions included the use of ARVs for Pre-Exposure Prophylaxis (PrEP) with either systemic use of drugs to high-risk subpopulations, or as localized intravaginal microbicides [34, 35]. At the same time, some advocated the use of HAART in all HIV-infected adults as a way of reducing transmission as well as treatment for disease [36, 37]. While such an approach should be effective if accompanied by widespread testing to identify as many HIV-positive people as possible, it seemed to be prohibitively expensive. At a time of global economic depression in the affluent countries, many agencies were questioning the sustainability of ARVs at current treatment levels in the developing world.

These observations were coming at a time when there was increasing optimism that ARVs could also be used to prevent transmissions in adults. Vaginal microbicides with ARVs like tenofovir showed protective benefit, and PrEP studies hold great promise [34, 35] (see Table 1.2).

Targeting the Transmitters

The highest VLs are observed during acute infection [41, 42] and years later when AIDS-defining illness is present and T-lymphocyte counts are falling rapidly. Acute and early infection has also been associated with the highest rates of transmission, because high blood VL is associated with high VL in reproductive tract fluids. Also, recently infected individuals are less likely to know they are infected as compared to those who have become ill after several years of infection, and they are more likely to feel healthy enough for sexual activity. Studies with discordant couples and other at-risk populations have shown a quantifiable increase in transmission associated with each increase in VL [43].

Table 1.2 Biomedical research approaches to prevention of HIV/AIDS

Category	Results	Comments	Reference
Vaccine	Generally poor	One recent design gave borderline efficacy, highly efficacious vaccine unlikely for at least a decade	Rerks-Ngarm et al. [38]
Treatment of venereal Herpes	No benefit	Control of Herpes replication in coinfected individuals gave no benefit in reducing transmission of HIV	Celum et al. [14]
Male circumcision	50–60% protection	Randomized controlled trials showed clear efficacy. Inexpensive	Quinn [12]
Microbicides-broad spectrum disinfectants	No benefit	Some even showed increased risk for infection, presumably through damage to mucosal surfaces	Balzarini and Van Damme [11]
Microbicides-antiretroviral (ARV) drugs	Some benefit	Vaginal Tenofovir gel gave 39% protection in recent trial	Abdool Karim et al. [34]
Prevention mother-to-child transmission with ARV	Excellent	Three-drug combinations prevent virtually all transmissions during pregnancy, birth, and breastfeeding	Shapiro et al. [30]
Postexposure prophylaxis with ARV	Apparently excellent	Occupational exposures followed by rapid ARV appear effective but not based on randomized trials	Bouvet et al. [39]
Preexposure prophylaxis with ARV	Beneficial	Efficacy in men who had sex with men who adhered to ARV regimen	Grant et al. [35]
Test and treat with ARV	Beneficial	High efficacy in discordant couples trial; no results available at community level	Cohen et al. [40]

Recent studies by our group in Botswana revealed that up to one-third of recently infected people had VLs of ≥50,000 per ml of blood that were maintained for at least 6 months after seroconversion, and the median duration of the high VL in this group was 350 days [44, 45]. This invites the hypothesis that such individuals could be responsible, at least in part, for the very high prevalence rates of HIV that are seen in southern Africa. It also suggests the possibility that selectively targeting this subset of individuals could be particularly effective in a "test and treat" approach for prevention of new infections.

If a "test and treat" strategy were undertaken in a particular region or locale, and most sexually active adults agreed to be tested for VL, we estimate that a large proportion of potential transmitters could be eliminated from the transmission pool if they took HAART [45]. To identify such individuals with extended early high VL, particularly those who are not yet eligible for treatment based on disease criteria or low CD4 counts, it will be necessary to utilize VL tests rather than just antibody tests at routine voluntary testing and counseling centers. Dried blood spot (DBS) screens can be done with a finger prick, negating the need for phlebotomy at the first visit. The DBS tests may not be as sensitive for detecting small fluctuations, particularly low VL, as might be needed for evaluating early changes in drug resistance.

However, for the semi-quantitative detection of high VL associated with transmission, such as 50,000 or 100,000, the DBS screen seems appropriate.

Recently, a study in discordant couples evaluated antiretroviral treatment (ART) to the infected partner to determine whether this decreased transmission between adults [40]. All HIV-infected partners were given ART after they reached lower CD4 levels, but half of those in a higher CD4 range were also given ART to determine whether it would reduce transmission. Using only matched transmissions, where it could be verified that the uninfected partner became infected from the index case, transmissions were reduced by 96% in couples where the index case received ART. Evidence for linkage of the infections to the index case was established by comparing the sequence of the newly infecting virus to the sequence of the HIV in the infected partner.

Cost-Effectiveness

For various governments, foundations, and international agencies, a major concern is the sustainability of ART for AIDS patients in low-income countries. The effectiveness of the treatment has been established. Patients appear to have high rates of adherence to their medications [27] resulting in low rates of drug resistance [46]. If the cost of treatment is at least $500–1,000 per year, similar to the entire per capita income, patients on ART live for more than 20 years, and 10–25% of adults are infected (as is the case in most countries in southern Africa), it is easy to see how financial sustainability may be questioned. If, for example, deaths from HIV/AIDS are reduced by 75% through treatment, then the total number of HIV-infected adults will go up unless new infections are decreased by 75%.

The universal use of ART for all HIV-infected adults has been proposed by several groups as a strategy to prevent new infections [36, 37]. However, this strategy would increase the global cost by a large proportion, at least for a decade or more. A logical cost-effective alternative would be to selectively treat only those HIV-infected individuals with high VL [45], in addition to those who qualify based on AIDS-defining illness or low CD4 lymphocyte numbers. This subset, which corresponds to 20–30% of infected individuals with HIV-1C infections in southern Africa, also lose CD4 lymphocytes more rapidly than others, meaning that they would usually qualify for disease-based HAART in 1–3 years rather than 4–6 years, as would those with lower VLs. Concentrating "treatment for prevention" on those with "extended acute" high VL should thus be cost-effective within very few years, and cost-saving long before a "treatment for all" approach.

Conclusions

Research to develop an efficacious vaccine for HIV/AIDS has been disappointing. This has been particularly discouraging for sub-Saharan Africa, where HIV transmission has been much more prevalent. Rates have been especially high in southern

Africa, which has about one-third of the world's HIV infections in less than 2% of the world's population. ART for AIDS has been highly successful throughout the world. ARVs for PMTCT has also shown very high efficacy when three-drug combinations are used. Recently, ARVs have also shown interesting promise in microbicides and prevention of infection in men who have sex with men. We have proposed the use of ARVs for prevention in subpopulations of heterosexuals in southern Africa who have sustained high VL. Because this intervention would be limited to those most likely to transmit, who are also most likely to progress rapidly to disease, it should be more cost-effective than generalized treatment of all HIV-infected individuals.

References

1. Gottlieb MS, Schroff R, Schanker HM, Weisman JD, Fan PT, Wolf RA et al (1981) *Pneumocystis carinii* pneumonia and mucosal candidiasis in previously healthy homosexual men: evidence of a new acquired cellular immunodeficiency. New Engl J Med 205:1425–1431
2. Masur H, Michelis MA, Greene JB, Onorato I, Stouwe RA, Holzman RS et al (1981) An outbreak of community-acquired *Pneumocystis carinii* pneumonia: initial manifestation of cellular immune dysfunction. New Engl J Med 205:1431–1438
3. Siegal FP, Lopez C, Hammer GS, Brown AE, Kornfeld SJ, Gold J et al (1981) Severe acquired immunodeficiency in male homosexuals, manifested by chronic perianal ulcerative herpes simplex lesions. New Engl J Med 305:1439–1444
4. Centers for Disease Control Task Force on Kaposi's Sarcoma and Opportunistic Infections (1982) Epidemiologic aspects of the current outbreak of Kaposi's sarcoma and opportunistic infections. New Engl J Med 306:248–252
5. Davis KC, Horburgh CR Jr, Hasiba U, Schocket AL, Kirkpatrick CH (1983) Acquired immunodeficiency syndrome in a patient with hemophilia. Ann Intern Med 98:284–286
6. Curran JW, Lawrence DN, Jaffe H, Kaplan JE, Zyla LD, Chamberland M et al (1984) Acquired immunodeficiency syndrome (AIDS) associated with transfusions. New Engl J Med 310:69–75
7. Oleske J, Minnefor A, Cooper R Jr, Thomas K, dela Cruz A, Ahdieh H, Guerrero I, Joshi W, Desposito F (1983) Immune deficiency syndrome in children. JAMA 249:2345–2349
8. Clumeck N, Mascart-Lemone F, de Maubeuge J, Brenez D, Marcelis L (1983) Acquired immune deficiency syndrome in Black Africans. Lancet 1:642
9. Gallo RC, Salahuddin SZ, Popovic M, Shearer GM, Kaplan M, Haynes BF et al (1984) Frequent detection and isolation of cytopathic retroviruses (HTLV-III) from patients with AIDS and at risk for AIDS. Science 224:500–503
10. Barre-Sinoussi F, Chermann JC, Rey F, Nugeyre T, Chamaret S, Gruest J et al (1983) Isolation of a T-lymphotropic retrovirus from a patient at risk for acquired immune deficiency syndrome (AIDS). Science 220:868–871
11. Balzarini J, Van Damme L (2007) Microbicide drug candidates to prevent HIV infection. Lancet 369:787–797
12. Quinn TC (2007) Circumcision and HIV transmission. Curr Opin Infect Dis 20:33–38
13. Kapiga SH, Sam NE, Bang H, Ni Q, Ao TTH, Kiwelu I et al (2007) The role of Herpes simplex virus type 2 and other genital infections in the acquisition of HIV-1 among high-risk women in northern Tanzania. J Infect Dis 195:1260–1269
14. Celum C, Wald A, Lingappa JR, Magaret AS, Wang RS, Mugo N et al (2010) Acyclovir and transmission of HIV-1 from persons infected with HIV-1 and HSV-2. New Engl J Med 362:427–439

15. UNAIDS (2010) Global report: UNAIDS report on the global AIDS epidemic. UNAIDS, Geneva. http://www.unaids.org
16. Gregson S, Gonese E, Hallett TB, Taruberekera N, Hargrove JW, Lopman B et al (2010) HIV decline in Zimbabwe due to reductions in risky sex? Evidence from a comprehensive epidemiological review. Int J Epidemiol 39:1311–1323
17. Essex M (2009) Clades, subtypes, strains, recombination and reinfection: clinical and epidemiological relevance. In: Kanki PJ, Marlink RG (eds) A line drawn in the sand. Harvard University Press, Cambridge, pp 245–258
18. Montano M, Nixon C, Ndung'u T, Bussman H, Novitsky VA, Dickman D et al (2000) Elevated TNFα activation of human immunodeficiency virus type 1 subtype C in southern Africa associated with a NFκB enhancer gain-of-function. J Infect Dis 181:76–81
19. Tscherning C, Alaeus A, Fredriksson R, Björndal Å, Deng H, Littman DR et al (1998) Differences in chemokine coreceptor usage between genetic subtypes of HIV-1. Virology 241:181–188
20. Cohen MS, Hellmann N, Levy JA, DeCock K, Lange J (2008) The spread, treatment, and prevention of HIV-1: evolution of a global pandemic. J Clin Invest 118:1244–1254
21. Essex M, Renjifo B, Peña-Cruz V, McLane MF, Marlink R, Lee TH et al (1997) Different subtypes of HIV-1 and cutaneous dendritic cells. Science 278:787–788
22. Pilcher CD, Tien HC, Eron JJ Jr, Vernazza PL, Leu SY, Stewart PW et al (2004) Brief but efficient: acute HIV infection and the sexual transmission of HIV. J Infect Dis 189:1785–1792
23. Neilson JR, John GC, Carr JK, Lewis P, Kreiss JK, Jackson S et al (1999) Subtypes of human immunodeficiency virus type 1 and disease stage among women in Nairobi, Kenya. J Virol 73:4393–4403
24. Centlivre M, Sala M, Wain-Hobson S, Berkhout B (2007) In HIV-1 pathogenesis the die is cast during primary infection. AIDS 21:1–11
25. Hirsch MS (1990) Chemotherapy of human immunodeficiency virus infections: current practice and future. J Infect Dis 161:845–857
26. Connor EM, Sperling RS, Gelber R, Kiselev P, Scott G, O'Sullivan MJ et al (1994) Reduction of maternal–infant transmission of human immunodeficiency virus type 1 with zidovudine treatment. New Engl J Med 331:1173–1180
27. Wester CW, Bussmann H, Koethe J, Moffat C, Vermund S, Essex M et al (2009) Adult combination antiretroviral therapy in sub-Saharan Africa: lessons from Botswana and future challenges. HIV Ther 3:501–526
28. Guay L, Musoke P, Fleming T, Bagenda D, Allen M, Nakabiito C et al (1999) Intrapartum and neonatal single-dose nevirapine compared with zidovudine for prevention of mother-to-child transmission of HIV-1 in Kampala, Uganda: HIVNET 012 randomised trial. Lancet 354:795–802
29. Lallemant M, Jourdain G, Le Coeur S, Mary JY, Ngo-Giang-Huong N, Koetsawang S et al (2004) Single-dose perinatal nevirapine plus standard zidovudine to prevent mother-to-child transmission of HIV-1 in Thailand. New Engl J Med 351:217–228
30. Shapiro RL, Hughes MD, Ogwu A, Kitch D, Lockman S, Moffat C et al (2010) Antiretroviral regimens in pregnancy and breast-feeding in Botswana. New Engl J Med 362:2282–2294
31. Thior I, Lockman S, Smeaton LM, Shapiro RL, Wester C, Heymann SJ et al (2006) Breastfeeding plus infant zidovudine prophylaxis for 6 months vs formula feeding plus infant zidovudine for 1 month to reduce mother-to-child HIV transmission in Botswana. A randomized trial: the Mashi study. JAMA 296:794–805
32. Shapiro RL, Ndung'u T, Lockman S, Smeaton LM, Thior I, Wester C et al (2005) Highly active antiretroviral therapy started during pregnancy or postpartum suppresses HIV-1 RNA, but not DNA, in breast milk. J Infect Dis 192:713–719
33. Koulinska IN, Villamor E, Chaplin B, Msamanga G, Fawzi W, Renjifo B et al (2006) Transmission of cell-free and cell-associated HIV-1 through breast-feeding. J Acquir Immune Defic Syndr 41:93–99

34. Abdool Karim Q, Abdool Karim SS, Frohlich JA, Grobler AC, Baxter C, Mansoor LE et al (2010) Effectiveness and safety of tenofovir gel, an antiretroviral microbicide, for the prevention of HIV infection in women. Science 329:1168–1174

35. Grant RM, Lama JR, Anderson PL, McMahan V, Liu AY, Vargas L et al (2010) Preexposure chemoprophylaxis for HIV prevention in men who have sex with men. New Engl J Med 363:2587–2599

36. Anema A, Wood E, Montaner JSG (2008) Medicine and society: the use of highly active retroviral therapy to reduce HIV incidence at the population level. CAJ 179:13–14

37. Granich RM, Gilks CF, Dye C, De Cock KM, Williams BG (2009) Universal voluntary HIV testing with immediate antiretroviral therapy as a strategy for elimination of HIV transmission: a mathematical model. Lancet 373:48–57

38. Rerks-Ngarm S, Pitisuttithum P, Nitayaphan S, Kaewkungwal J, Chiu J, Paris R et al (2009) Vaccination with ALVAC and AIDSVAX to prevent HIV-1 infection in Thailand. New Engl J Med 361:2209–2220

39. Bouvet E, Laporte A, Tarantola A (2002) Postexposure prophylaxis for occupational exposure and sexual assault. In: Essex M, Mboup S, Kanki P, Marlink R, Tlou S (eds) AIDS in Africa, 2nd edn. Kluwer Academic/Plenum, New York, p 571

40. Cohen MS, Chen YQ, McCauley M, Gamble T, Hosseinipour MC, Kumarasamy N et al (2011) Prevention of HIV-1 infection with early antiretroviral therapy. New Engl J Med 365: 493–505

41. Fideli US, Allen SA, Musonda R, Trask S, Hahn BH, Weiss H et al (2001) Virologic and immunologic determinants of heterosexual transmission of human immunodeficiency virus type 1 in Africa. AIDS Res Hum Retrovir 17:901–910

42. Wawer MJ, Gray RH, Sewankambo NK, Serwadda D, Xianbin L, Laeyendecker O et al (2005) Rates of HIV-1 transmission per coital act, by stage of HIV-1 infection, in Rakai, Uganda. J Infect Dis 191:1403–1409

43. Lingappa JR, Hughes JP, Wang RS, Baeten JM, Celum C, Gray GE et al (2010) Estimating the impact of plasma HIV-1 RNA reductions on heterosexual HIV-1 transmission risk. PLoS One 5:e12598

44. Novitsky V, Wang R, Bussmann H, Lockman S, Baum M, Shapiro R et al (2010) HIV-1 subtype C infected individuals maintaining high viral load as potential targets for the "test-and-treat" approach to reduce HIV transmission. PLoS One 5:e10148

45. Novitsky V, Ndung'u T, Wang R, Bussmann H, Chonco F, Makhema J et al (2011) Extended high viremics: a substantial fraction of individuals maintain high plasma viral RNA levels after acute HIV-1 subtype C infection. AIDS 25:1515–1522

46. Bussmann H, Novitsky V, Wester W, Peter T, Masupu K, Gabaitiri L et al (2005) HIV-1 subtype C drug resistance background among ARV-naïve adults in Botswana. Antivir Chem Chemother 16:103–115

Chapter 2
Study Report on Prevention of Mother-to-Child Transmission for HIV-Infected Pregnant Women in Yunnan Province*

Zengquan Zhou, Kathrine Meyers, Qingling Chen, Yunfei Lao, and Haoyu Qian

Introduction

Yunnan Province is the origins and heartland of China's AIDS epidemic. While the epidemic was for many years concentrated among injecting drug users, over the past few years it can be characterized as an epidemic driven as much by sexual transmission. Sixty-four percent of newly identified cases in 2009 are attributable to hetero and homosexual transmission [1]. With increased sexual transmission naturally comes the increased risk of vertical transmission from mother to baby in utero, during labor and delivery, or through breastfeeding. In 2009, 1.5% of newly reported cases were cases of mother-to-child transmission (MTCT) [1]. The national and provincial governments have invested heavily to combat the spread of the AIDS epidemic in Yunnan, initially with a focus on harm reduction programs for drug users and in more recent years extending the work to other populations and transmission routes as well. In 2003, the national prevention of mother-to-child transmission

*The projects on which this research is based were supported by Elizabeth Glaser Pediatric AIDS Foundation, Gracious Glory Buddhism Foundation, Rotary International, Tai Foundation, ZeShan Foundation, and other contributions from Kevin Tang, Oscar Tang, Shirley and Walter Wang, and Miranda Wong Tang.

Z. Zhou, M.D. (✉)
Yunnan AIDS Care Center, Xiuyuan Road, Xishan District,
Kunming, Yunnan, China

Yunnan AIDS Initiative, Kunming, China
e-mail: ynzzq@263.net

K. Meyers, Dr.P.H. • H. Qian, M.P.H.
Aaron Diamond AIDS Research Center, 455 1st Avenue #7, New York, NY 10016, USA

Q. Chen, M.D. • Y. Lao, M.P.H.
Yunnan AIDS Care Center, Xiuyuan Road, Xishan District,
Kunming, Yunnan, China
e-mail: ynzzq@263.net

Y. Lu et al. (eds.), *HIV/AIDS Treatment in Resource Poor Countries: Public Health Challenges*, DOI 10.1007/978-1-4614-4520-3_2,
© Springer Science+Business Media New York 2013

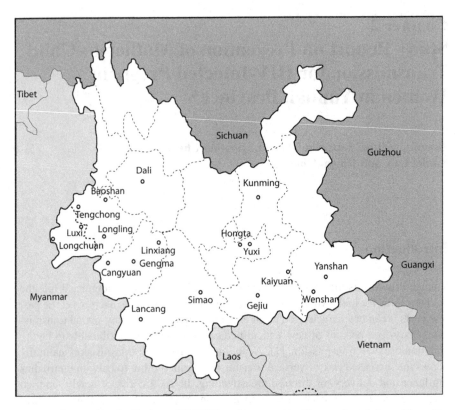

Fig. 2.1 Geographic distribution of PMTCT project counties. Figure adapted from: Zhou, Z, Meyers, K, Li, X, et al. (2010). Prevention of mother-to-child transmission of HIV-1 using highly active antiretroviral therapy in rural Yunnan, China. *Journal of Acquired Immune Deficiency Syndromes*, 53(Supplement), S15–S22

(PMTCT) program was piloted in two Yunnan counties. Three years later all 129 counties in Yunnan were covered in the national PMTCT program that recommended and provided azidothymidine (AZT) starting at 28 weeks gestation plus single-dose nevirapine (sdNVP) during labor and delivery for the mother and neonate, a protocol that in combination with safe feeding practices can bring transmission rate as low as 1.8% according to one study [2], although with risks of inducing drug resistance for women who may later require treatment for their own disease. In practice, because many women are identified as HIV infected only when they present at the clinic in labor, the use of sdNVP, associated with a 10.8% transmission rate [3], is still highly prevalent. In the national PMTCT program, infants are diagnosed by antibody test after 18 months of age when maternal antibodies are no longer present in the child's blood. Twelve months of formula feeding are provided as well.

In this context, in 2005 the Aaron Diamond AIDS Research Center (ADARC) in partnership with the Yunnan Province Bureau of Health launched a demonstration project to test the safety, effectiveness, and feasibility of providing highly active antiretroviral therapy (HAART) for HIV-infected pregnant women to interrupt HIV transmission to their infants in 18 counties in Yunnan (Fig. 2.1). The following year the Elizabeth Glaser Pediatric AIDS Foundation (EGPAF) joined these efforts and provided an additional 3 years of support to develop a model of PMTCT that expanded out from the mainly clinical focus to take on a more comprehensive public health approach. The program has since expanded to 132 township and county facilities in eight counties. The provincial AIDS treatment authority, the Yunnan AIDS Care Center and a Kunming-based NGO, the Yunnan AIDS Initiative have been tasked with implementation of the program. Finally, in 2009, with support from Hong Kong's Zeshan Foundation, the program added an additional component to integrate screening and PMTCT of hepatitis B virus (HBV) infection and syphilis with HIV in six counties to explore the feasibility of packaged testing as a part of standard antenatal care (ANC) services.

Program Design

Mobilization of Leaders

Local leadership support and buy-in are critical in the increasingly decentralized system of governance that has developed in China since opening and reform began in 1978. In the context of a complex public health intervention like PMTCT, "local" captures multiple tiers of administration and bureaucracy across multiple sectors. Key leaders include Bureau of Health administrators at the provincial, prefecture, and county levels; administrators of all health facilities participating in the program; administrators from the prefecture and county centers for disease prevention and control (CDC); township and village administrative leaders; and women leaders at all the program sites. The support of all these individuals does not only have to be built at the onset of the program but also must be maintained over time. Over the course of 6 years, leaders often get promoted or demoted, or they change sectors entirely, thereby requiring investment of time and resources by the program team into advocacy across the life of the program.

Establishment and Strengthening of PMTCT Network

Across most of Yunnan, the county is the lowest level on the administrative hierarchy able to provide HIV/AIDS services from testing to ARV (antiretroviral) treatment, including PMTCT interventions. Administratively this makes sense, as the number of HIV-infected cases distributed in each county is not overwhelmingly large. However, Yunnan's mountainous terrain and underdeveloped road infrastructure make access to county health facilities very challenging for the majority of rural residents. Their most regular point of contact with the health system is at the township and village level.

To address this critical access issue our program sought to build the capacity of township and village level health workers to take over critical elements of PMTCT services, and to form close vertical linkages with the county-level maternal child health (MCH) clinic. At the same time, the program also stressed the need for strong horizontal referrals between the MCH and the CDC and hospitals for laboratory tests and follow-up of HIV-positive women beyond their perinatal period.

Improving HIV Counseling and Testing

Improving the quality and reach of counseling and testing was a focal point of the program. Yunnan policy demands universal screening of pregnant women and premarital couples and this provides the critical regulatory basis of our work. Our program sought to overcome the implementation challenges in carrying out this directive, and to ensure that the services provided were effective vehicles for promoting HIV prevention education for the 99% of women who remain uninfected. The specific areas we worked on include: expanded coverage of counseling and testing out from county health facilities to township and village level; improved HIV counseling of all pregnant women at ANC and labor and delivery; improved coordination of the MCH with the civil affairs bureau so that all premarital registrants will be counseled and tested for HIV.

Optimal PMTCT Services for HIV Pregnant Women

In the USA and Europe, vertical transmission has been virtually eliminated with HAART-based PMTCT regimens. The effectiveness of perinatal ARV prophylaxis, safe delivery methods, and formula feeding in reducing rate of MTCT from 30% to 40% down to less than 2% has been thoroughly demonstrated [4]. A primary program objective was to demonstrate that even though rural Yunnan is a resource-limited setting, it was possible to deliver interventions according to international standards, and achieve results comparable to developed nations. Together the Yunnan Health Bureau and ADARC set out to demonstrate the feasibility, safety, and efficacy of HAART prophylaxis for PMTCT at our project sites, with the hope that the results can be used to advocate for the adaptation of this project model across China.

Continued Care and Support for HIV-Positive Women and Families

Yunnan HIV/AIDS guidelines state that after pregnancy, HIV-infected women who do not require HAART should be referred to the CDC for follow-up, and women who reach treatment criteria shall be referred to the county comprehensive hospital for

HAART treatment. This program not only provided technical support to the MCH hospitals, but also worked closely with the CDC and the comprehensive hospitals to facilitate the linkage between PMTCT and care and treatment. In addition, we provided support for each program county to establish positive women and family support groups as a platform for women and their families to share their experiences and provide mutual support. Doctors could also use these positive support group meetings as opportunities to reinforce various health knowledge and practices, such as adherence to ARV therapy and infant feeding support.

Method

County and Facility Site Selection

Sites were selected based on HIV-1 prevalence among ANC clients, existing HAART services at the county hospital, and some experience in PMTCT interventions. Among the 18 sites selected, 13 were county-level MCH clinics, 4 were prefectural-level MCH clinics, and 1 was a municipal MCH clinic in the provincial capital of Kunming. HIV prevalence rate among the pregnant women population at the 18 sites ranged from 0.4% to 2% enrollment began at five sites in 2005, nine more in 2006, two in 2008, and two more in 2009. Half of the counties are designated poverty counties by the national and provincial governments, and seven counties have an average per capita income of less than $1 a day.

In addition to selecting geographic sites, we selected specific facilities in which to push services out to the periphery. Specifically, after EGPAF joined the program in 2007, we selected townships with the highest number of cases as focal points in which to invest in the capacity-building of village doctors and township hospitals to identify pregnant women early in gestation, provide basic HIV and PMTCT information, and either provide HIV rapid test to pregnant women in the village, or refer them to the township health center for HIV testing. At the township level, we worked with the MCH system to distribute HIV rapid test kits at all the township health centers and integrate HIV counseling and testing as a routine part of ANC and labor and delivery services.

Enrollment into Clinical Program

Eligibility criteria for pregnant women to be enrolled into the program to receive HAART prophylaxis were the following: they planned to deliver their babies; they were able to give written informed consent; and they did not intend to move outside the county during the pregnancy period. Women not enrolled met one or more of the following exclusion criteria: serious opportunistic infection or AIDS-related tumor; abnormal liver or renal function; co-infected with hepatitis B or C virus;

severe anemia, thrombocytopenia, and leukopenia; serious risk of other pregnancy complication; acute or chronic pancreatitis; alcohol or drug addiction; and serious psychiatric illness. Those who did not meet the qualifications were enrolled into the government PMTCT program.

Intervention

All women received HAART, beginning as early as the 14th week of pregnancy. Planned C-sections were recommended if the duration of HAART was short or viral load late in pregnancy was high. Neonates were given sdNVP within 24 h of birth and 1 week of AZT if the mother had been on treatment for more than 4 weeks at the time of labor. Otherwise, neonates were given 4 weeks of AZT. Parents were counseled to formula-feed their baby exclusively, and follow-up visits were scheduled at 1 week, 1 month and once a month thereafter, and immediately in the event of any health problems.

Dry blood spots (DBS) from HIV-exposed infants were collected in each project county. Samples were shipped through the postal service at room temperature to the Yunnan AIDS Care Center laboratory, which has been certified to perform DNA PCR. Genomic DNA was isolated from DBS by extraction using a polyvalent cationic resin, chelex 100 (Biorad, Marnes-la-Coquette, Paris, France). HIV-1 DNA (gag, pol and env gp41 regions) was detected by two rounds of PCR amplification.

Women with CD4 counts above $350/mm^3$ at enrollment discontinued treatment after delivery, unless their CD4 had fallen below $350/mm^3$. These women were referred to the county CDC for regular follow-up. Women with CD4 counts below $350/mm^3$ at enrollment were referred to the local government-designated ARV treatment hospital 6 weeks postdelivery to continue treatment.

Key Lessons and Results

Sustained Advocacy at Multiple Levels

Our leadership advocacy efforts focused first on the Yunnan Provincial Bureau of Health. At this level, it was beneficial to have internationally well-known experts such as Dr. David Ho, Director of the Aaron Diamond AIDS Research Center, at meetings with provincial Bureau of Health leadership to explain the significance of the program, and its potential contribution to overall HIV/AIDS prevention and treatment in Yunnan. The provincial Bureau of Health recognized the significance of the program very quickly and at program initiation gathered all the heads of prefecture to sign official program responsibility documents.

The next step was the integration of a leadership advocacy component into our trainings at each level. In addition to the health providers who directly provide PMTCT services, we required county Bureau of Health, MCH and hospital administrators to attend nontechnical parts of the trainings designed to raise their awareness of the importance of PMTCT, and empower them to take on responsibility of local PMTCT work from a management perspective. Even though the government had designated HIV prevention and treatment work, including PMTCT, as a priority, many local leaders did not see HIV as a significant concern in their area. Many of them confessed to coming into our training with the intention of sleeping through it. However, through our continued effort, these leaders grew to appreciate the significance of PMTCT in the context of HIV and women and children's health, and to see the program as an opportunity to strengthen their local health system.

Finally, leadership advocacy requires sustained efforts. Throughout the program, we maintained close communication with county administrators whenever we traveled to counties on site visits. The administrators were invited to program conferences so they could be updated on program progress and participate in planning and implementation of next steps. Leadership changes occurred frequently throughout the life of the program. It was critical to learn of these changes as quickly as possible so that we could inform the new administrators of the program and secure their support.

Improved Quality and Coverage of HIV Counseling and Testing

While the efficacy of interventions to reduce the rate of vertical transmission is extremely high, the critical first step is the identification of HIV-positive pregnant women. Expanding counseling and testing coverage to capture women who are not seen at county health facilities was therefore an instrumental component of our program strategy.

The first challenge was to build up capacity of township and village health workers to provide high-quality counseling and testing services. We developed a training curriculum targeted to rural community level health workers. Most township and village doctors have no higher than a vocational high school education. While most of them had heard about HIV/AIDS through the media and through half-day training sessions administered by government health agencies, these trainings were pedagogically uninspired: usually monotonous in both style and method, with one person lecturing in front to a hall full of attendees. Our training curriculum was adapted from the USCDC PMTCT curriculum, with a strong emphasis on HIV counseling, as that was the area we felt community health workers would be most directly involved. Each of our training workshops was limited to 40 people to facilitate the use of participatory training and learning methods. Workshops were usually 2 days in length, and we used a mixture of training methods including slide presentations, demonstrations, role-plays, games and activities, discussion groups, and videos. This integrated approach was not only effective in knowledge transfer but also facilitated the acquisition of practical skills, and promoted attitudinal change. For most village and township health workers, our training was a completely novel experience.

Trainees expressed that they had never known that trainings could be so informative and yet fun at the same time. Through our trainings, health providers noted that they became more confident at providing HIV counseling and testing. They also embraced participatory training methods that they have now adapted for use in public education events in their townships and villages.

Through these trainings, the program successfully increased coverage of HIV counseling and testing in rural areas. The number of pregnant women who received counseling and testing at township health centers more than doubled from 16,057 in 2007 to 36,791 in 2009. Also, 249 village doctors trained by our program have started to provide HIV rapid testing at their village clinics, which is unique in all of China. The expansion of counseling and testing services out to the peripheral areas has translated directly into increase in coverage rates for HIV testing of pregnant women. HIV testing coverage increased from 46% of all pregnant women in 2005 to 95% of pregnant women at all the sites in 2009.

The program also supported HIV counseling and testing of premarital couples. Marriage licensing is under the jurisdiction of the Civil Affairs Bureau, while the responsibility for HIV counseling and testing in this population lies with the MCH. In our project counties, the MCH coordinated with the local Civil Affairs Department either to set up counseling and testing windows at the marriage registration office, or to set up a referral system to the MCH for registrants. Gradually, HIV counseling and testing for premarital couples has also expanded out to the township health clinics in order to reach those rural couples who do not go to the county for registration.

Improved Clinical Services for PMTCT

An ARV regimen for HIV-infected pregnant women represents a critical component of comprehensive PMTCT interventions. Our work to improve early testing of pregnant women and early identification of positive women allowed our program to start more women on complex regimens earlier during their pregnancy.

When our program first started, health workers within the MCH lacked both knowledge and experience in the administration of ARVs, which were the purview of infectious disease doctors at specifically designated hospitals. Given the novelty of PMTCT in China in 2005, often the first advice given to HIV-infected pregnant women was to terminate their pregnancy. For those who chose to continue their pregnancy, it was common for providers to only prescribe sdNVP during labor and delivery, even if the woman was identified as HIV-infected earlier in her pregnancy. Gradually some MCH doctors began to provide scAZT prophylaxis during pregnancy, which marked a significant step forward. However, most MCH health providers neither had sufficient understanding of the importance of CD4 testing and clinical staging, nor the capacity to perform CD4 test or staging at the MCH hospital. The most they could do was to refer patients to the CDC for further testing; however in the early years of China's PMTCT program very few referrals were completed, thus missing a great opportunity to link up PMTCT with care and treatment.

Technical support has focused on two areas to bolster the effectiveness and safety of optimal prophylactic intervention. One is to link up the MCH and its doctors with the ARV treatment system, both with the local comprehensive hospital's infectious disease clinic and with the provincial body responsible for overseeing treatment, the Yunnan provincial AIDS Care Center (YACC). At the same time, we provided training and continuous support to the MCH obstetricians and pediatricians themselves to raise their confidence and skill levels in managing HAART prophylaxis for HIV-infected pregnant women.

Process indicators collected suggest that over time, implementation of the project has improved. First, the pace of enrollment of women into the HAART regimen in each county increased over the years. During the first 3 years of enrollment, a total of 88 women received HAART; in 2008 and 2009, 181 women who delivered during these 2 years received HAART prophylaxis; and in 2010 alone, 121 women have been enrolled. Discussions with project staff and doctors reveal that they attribute this increase in enrollment to earlier identification of HIV-infected pregnant women and greater confidence in their own skills. The early reluctance in treating HIV-infected pregnant women with HAART has been turned into firm belief in HAART prophylaxis as the best option for PMTCT. As they learn to manage HAART for women, and more and more HIV-free babies are born to HIV-positive mothers under their care, not only have they become more confident in themselves but also HIV-positive women come to trust that they can lead healthy lives and have healthy babies under the doctors' care. Many doctors recalled how difficult it was to follow-up with women in the first years of the program, but now most women actively seek the doctor's counsel, and adhere well to their follow-up schedule.

The 390 women who have received HAART prophylaxis gave birth to 395 babies, including five sets of twins. A total of three babies have become infected with HIV-1 in this cohort, an infection rate of 0.76%.

In addition to our technical guidance to strengthen linkages between PMTCT and treatment, and our training of health providers at the MCH system, the financial support provided through the program fills resource gaps for necessary examinations and tests to closely monitor the health of the women on HAART. Our program ensured that standard blood work and physical examination were performed for the women at start of HAART and at regular intervals throughout their pregnancy. In addition, blood was drawn to measure CD4 counts and viral loads at the start of treatment, at labor and delivery, and at 1, 3, 6, and 12 months after initiation of HAART. Sixty-five percent of the women had an undetectable viral load at the time of delivery, demonstrating the effectiveness of HAART as a prophylaxis. We also closely monitored for adverse effects in the women using HAART prophylaxis. While 37% of women reported some type of adverse reaction, most were short-term, light adverse reactions. Twelve women switched to an alternate regimen, no women discontinued treatment due to side effects, and all mothers in the cohort remain alive.

Overall, 49% of the women had CD4 counts less than 350/mm^3 at the start of HAART prophylaxis and continued on treatment after delivery. This underscores another important advantage of starting women on HAART for PMTCT: linkage to treatment can be established using PMTCT as an entry point.

Introduction of Early Infant Diagnostics

Standard practice in China for infant diagnostics is ELISA testing of HIV-exposed infants at 12 months, followed by another ELISA confirmation at 18 months. With technical support from ADARC, we developed the capacity of the laboratory at Yunnan AIDS Care Center to perform DNA-PCR for HIV-exposed infants as early as 6 weeks. As the laboratory technique became reliable, more and more exposed infants were tested using DNA-PCR. Since we introduced early infant diagnostics (EID) at our program site in 2006, 428 HIV-exposed infants were tested using EID, which included not only infants of mothers enrolled into HAART prophylaxis, but of mothers enrolled into the national program as well. We have seen that the age of the babies for when the blood sample for DBS was collected has been significantly reduced as the program progresses. Among the 22 babies for whom we have test date in 2006 and 2007, the mean age of babies at blood draw was 109 days. Among 95 babies tested in 2008 and 2009, the mean age of babies was 59 days.

Strengthened Health Network

The significant results we achieved in expanding early screening of pregnant women and improving PMTCT prophylaxis to reduce the rate of MTCT would not have been possible without strengthening the local health network as a whole. In order to strengthen health system networks, it was necessary to first raise local health workers' and administrators' awareness on the importance of close collaboration between the sectors. When PMTCT work first started, many health providers held a rather limited view of PMTCT as providing prophylaxis for HIV-positive women who desired to have the baby, delivering babies by C-section, and providing them with formula provided by the government. Through the program, we gradually introduced a more comprehensive approach to PMTCT. Using the WHO (World Health Organization) PMTCT 4 components as a basis, we advocated for a comprehensive approach of PMTCT using "three preventions and one care"; that is, primary prevention, secondary prevention, prevention of MTCT, and care and treatment for positive women and families.

At the project's inception many health administrators and providers were concerned about the feasibility and necessity of implementing PMTCT services in such a comprehensive way. They understood that if a HIV-positive woman wanted to have the baby, then it was their responsibility to provide her and her baby with prophylaxis, deliver her baby at the hospital, and provide formula to feed the baby. But the idea of providing HIV counseling to every woman at ANC and labor and delivery, expanding counseling and testing service out to the township and village level where many doctors had nothing higher than a high school degree and no previous experience, giving HAART to women which would require close clinical and lab monitoring throughout the pregnancy, was daunting. There was also widespread concern that if the MCH was going to lead such a systematic effort, the stigma associated with AIDS would negatively impact the overall operation of the hospital. Fortunately, such fears turned out to be unfounded.

Instead, PMTCT program support for the county MCH enabled them to strengthen its network at the township hospital and village level, and led to improvements in rates of hospital deliveries, and strengthening of child immunization coverage. The various components worked in synergy: government-supported initiatives such as the new rural cooperative medical scheme assisted our efforts to improve PMTCT service provision, and our project also facilitated implementation of government-supported work in improving women and children's health. In fact, after a couple of years of our program, we could see that many of our MCH hospital sites showed significant increase in their in-hospital delivery rates each year. Many of the health administrators at the county MCH hospitals expressed that the biggest asset of the program was that it enabled them to strengthen their connection to the township level health centers and bolster their ties with the county hospital and CDC. With those strengthened networks, they will be able to provide better services in the future even without program support.

Integrating Screening and Prophylaxis for Multiple Vertically Transmitted Diseases

Building upon the foundation of the HIV PMTCT program, we saw an opportunity and the need to integrate HBV and syphilis screening with HIV screening at ANC and labor and delivery. Between January and August 2009, over 13,000 pregnant women received HIV, HBV, and syphilis counseling and testing at 12 prefecture and county-level health facilities in a pilot project. Of all the infants born of HBV surface antigen-positive mothers, 266 were immunized according to Chinese Medical Association guidelines (three shots over first 6 months of life), with an additional single hepatitis B immunoglobulin (HBIG) shot within 24 h of birth. Thirty-four syphilis-positive women received benzathine penicillin treatment regimen before their delivery. In addition, partners of HBV- or syphilis-infected women were also offered counseling, testing, and follow-up services.

Our pilot project demonstrated that the acceptance rate for testing and intervention was quite high. Packaging the three tests greatly improves the cost-effectiveness of ANC services and should be beneficial for a country like China, where prevalence of HBV is 7.2% among the general population and syphilis infection rate has risen steadily in recent years [5, 6].

Positive Support Groups

Mood disorders among PLWHA (people living with HIV/AIDS) such as anxiety and depression have been well documented in the literature [7, 8]. Psychosocial care and support is important for HIV-positive women to help them overcome their feelings of anxiety, fear, and despair. To meet their needs, our program developed psychosocial support groups for HIV-positive women and their families at all of our county MCH clinics. The meetings of the groups have served as venues for women to provide each other with mutual support, and for doctors to reinforce medical information and provide referrals to other resources available in the community.

Since 2007, 13 support groups from our sites have met close to 200 times. Spouses and other family members also actively participated in the support group meetings. Participants express some measure of relief from the isolation and loneliness they feel in their daily lives. The group meetings offer a forum for women to articulate their thoughts and concerns to others who have gone through or are going through similar experiences and emotions. Whenever possible we have tried to build the capacity of one or two women in the group to act as peer facilitators, as it seems that women more readily accept and absorb information shared by a peer rather than by a healthcare provider.

Support groups, with the patient's consent, have made specific efforts to involve partners and other family members. Support from family members is important for any person living with HIV, especially for HIV-infected pregnant women, where spousal support for treatment during pregnancy and infant feeding is critical. In rural China, where many young married couples live with the parents of the husband, the involvement of the mother-in-law in the support groups has proven especially beneficial. Through their participation these older women learn about HIV generally, and more importantly, witness the health and vitality of mothers and infants who have undergone the PMTCT intervention. Partners' and family members' support can contribute to a more supportive and harmonious atmosphere in the home. Overall, our support groups serve as a platform for providing HIV-infected women psychosocial support, promoting improved relationship with their family members, and acting as a complimentary force to clinical treatment.

Challenges and Next Steps

Infant Feeding Practices for HIV-Exposed Babies

High mortality rates among HIV-exposed, uninfected children have been observed and studied in a diverse range of settings [9–13]. Many of these deaths are associated with infant feeding practices [9–13]. The national and provincial PMTCT program in China generously provide 12 months of infant formula to all HIV-exposed babies with the assumption that as long as the formula is made available, babies will be protected from exposure to HIV through breast milk and will survive and thrive.

In 2008, we began to gather preliminary evidence of deaths among HIV-exposed babies in six counties. The data suggested higher mortality rates in HIV-exposed infants compared to the general population of infants in the same geographic areas.

Analyzing the causes of death, we found that up to 53% of them were potentially related to feeding or nutrition issues like diarrhea and malnutrition.

Sharing these preliminary findings with our county sites, we worked together to adapt a WHO/PATH (Program for Appropriate Technology in Health) curriculum on infant feeding and follow-up and used the curriculum in a training of prefecture and county-level physicians. The curriculum included the most up-to-date research on infant feeding practices, including studies that demonstrated the benefits of breastfeeding even for babies of HIV-infected mothers [14]. Through this awareness-building and skills-building exercise, health providers realized that in many rural areas environmental barriers to safe feeding practices are very high, even if free formula is being provided. They also admit that continued feeding counseling and support is a weak area in their work that can be improved upon.

Even though many doctors still find recommending and supporting of exclusive breastfeeding of HIV-exposed infants extremely challenging, they expressed willingness to explore this feeding option, as they had already been concerned with the sustainability of long-term government provision of 12 months of infant formula, as well as the safety issues of infant formula as exposed by the melamine scandal in recent years.

Our program is planning a pilot project in which we will strive to strengthen feeding counseling and support to HIV-positive mothers, regardless of the feeding option, at the same time explore breastfeeding for positive mothers who cannot meet safety requirements for formula feeding. We hope that health workers may gain experience and confidence in recommending exclusive breastfeeding while using ARV prophylaxis as a safe, viable option, and be able to provide effective support to these who choose to breastfeed.

Expansion of Program Model Still Needs Outside Support

We have demonstrated that a HAART regimen for PMTCT in a remote, resource-limited setting in China is feasible, and have achieved a reduction in MTCT rate comparable to that achieved in developed nations. We hold the conviction that from a standpoint of reducing MTCT and maximizing the mother's health, HAART is the best and the only choice for PMTCT and are heartened that the revised WHO guideline for PMTCT lists HAART prophylaxis as one option [15].

Even though rural China still lags in development compared to large metropolitan areas, given the vast rise in economic power of China on the world stage, and given the still very low overall prevalence of HIV, providing HAART for all pregnant woman and virtual elimination of MTCT should be an achievable and worthy goal. We hope our program efforts and results are only the beginning of nationwide effort to build up health infrastructure to provide comprehensive PMTCT services and to promote the use of optimal therapy for PMTCT intervention. In this regard, international organizations' participation in national-level advocacy, technical and financial assistance in systematic capacity building will remain critical.

Ongoing Capacity Building and Systems Strengthening Required

Through our project, we have helped the local health systems build a team of health providers capable of carrying out PMTCT services. However, rural health facility staffing remains very limited in general. There is no clear division between administrative and clinical responsibilities so that workloads for most doctors are heavy. While our program has promoted the integration of all PMTCT services into routine MCH work and we have seen significant progress in this regard, there are still many counties in which two or three doctors at the county level have sole or majority responsibility for all PMTCT services. We recommend the systematic distribution of PMTCT services should be further improved at health facilities, so that this work truly becomes a routine part of ANC, labor and delivery, and follow-up services and not the purview of one or two individual doctors.

Looking into the future regarding sustained implementation of PMTCT services at the community level, we feel that it will be critical to maintain training of health workers in order to reinforce the knowledge and skills, and to keep them updated on new information related to PMTCT.

Conclusion

While the primary endpoint of our PMTCT program has been achieved—fewer than 1% of HIV-exposed babies in our cohort have become infected in our program counties—the next step is to ensure that these results can be translated into a sustainable, province-wide model that can replicate these results and maximize HIV-free survival of exposed infants.

Nationally, the vertical transmission rate remains above 10% [16]. It is our hope that our experiences, as summarized in this chapter, may serve as building blocks from which the provincial and national PMTCT programs can extract key lessons and move toward decreased rates of MTCT and a generation of babies born free of HIV and surviving to lead productive, healthy lives.

Acknowledgments The authors wish to thank Dr. David Ho and Yunnan Bureau of Health Director Chen Juemin for their firm support of this program. We also thank the local project teams for their dedication and hard work, without which the successes described could never have been achieved. Finally, we extend our deep gratitude to all the women and their families who have entrusted us with their care and whose health and courage in the face of adversity inspire us daily.

References

1. Yunnan CDC (2010) Yunnan CDC annual report for HIV epidemic in 2009. Yunnan CDC, Kunming
2. Lallemant M, Conzague J, Le Coeur S et al (2004) Single-dose perinatal nevirapine plus standard zidovudine to prevent mother-to-child-transmission of HIV-1 in Thailand. New Engl J Med 351(3):217–228

3. Moodley D, Moodley J, Coovadia H et al (2003) A multicenter randomized controlled trial of nevirapine versus a combination of zidovudine and lamivudine to reduce intrapartum and early postpartum mother-to-child-transmission of HIV type 1. J Infect Dis 187(5):725–735
4. Volmink J, Siegfried NL, Merwe L et al (2007) Antiretrovirals for reducing the risk of mother-to-child transmission of HIV infection. Cochrane Database Syst Rev CD003510
5. Cohen MS, Hawkes S, Mabey D (2006) Syphilis returns to China ... with a vengeance. Sex Transmit Dis 33(12):724–725
6. Liang X, Bi S, Yang W et al (2009) Epidemiological serosurvey of hepatitis B in China—declining HBV prevalence due to hepatitis B vaccination. Vaccine 27(47):6550–6557
7. Kwalombota M (2002) The effect of pregnancy in HIV-infected women. AIDS Care 14(3): 431–433
8. Napravnik S, Royce R, Walter E, Lim W (2000) HIV-1 infected women and prenatal care utilization: barriers and facilitators. AIDS Patient Care STDs 14(8):411–420
9. Brahmbhatt H, Kigozi G, Wabwire-Mangen F et al (2006) Mortality in HIV-infected and uninfected children of HIV-infected and uninfected mothers in rural Uganda. J Acquir Immune Defic Syndr 41:504–508
10. Chilongozi D, Wang L, Brown L et al (2008) Morbidity and mortality among a cohort of human immunodeficiency virus type 1-infected and uninfected pregnant women and their infants from Malawi, Zambia, and Tanzania. Pediatr Infect Dis J 27(9):808–814
11. Marinda E, Humphrey JH, Iliff PJ et al (2007) Child mortality according to maternal and infant HIV status in Zimbabwe. Pediatr Infect Dis J 26(6):519–526
12. Newell M, Coovadia H, Cortina-Borja M et al (2004) Mortality of infected and uninfected infants born to HIV-infected mothers in Africa: a pooled analysis. Lancet 364(9441): 1236–1243
13. Shapiro R, Lockman S, Kim S et al (2007) Infant morbidity, mortality, and breast milk immunologic profiles among breastfeeding HIV-infected and HIV-uninfected women in Botswana. J Infect Dis 196(Supplement):S62–S69
14. Iliff P, Piwoz E, Tavengwa N et al (2005) Early exclusive breastfeeding reduces the risk of postnatal HIV-1 transmission and increases HIV-free survival. AIDS 19:699–708
15. WHO (2012) Programmatic update: use of antiretroviral drugs for treating pregnant women and preventing HIV infection in infants. WHO, Geneva. April 2012. http://www.who.int/hiv/PMTCT_update.pdf. Accessed August 20, 2012
16. Wang LH, Fang LW, Wang Q et al (2008) The rate and stages of HIV mother to child transmission in some areas of China with relatively high HIV/AIDS prevalence and evaluation of the effectiveness of relevant interventions. Chin J AIDS STD 14(5):435–438

Chapter 3
Antiretroviral Treatment Compliance in the Wenlou Village of Henan Province: A Case Study in Rural China

Xiaoduan Cheng

Patients, Clinics, and Available ARV Drugs

The village clinic is located inside the Wenlou village of the Lugang township in the Shangcai County of the Henan Province. The National Free antiretroviral (ARV) Treatment Program first started in this village as a pilot study in 2002. The program was fully launched the following year. Between September and December 2009, 271 AIDS patients from this clinic participated in this study. The oldest patient was 71 and youngest was 31 years old. There were 133 male and 138 female patients. Most of these patients (267 of 271) were infected through the plasma collection equipment contaminated with HIV-1 through the past poorly regulated commercial activities of selling blood in the previous decade. Two patients were infected by sexual intercourse, and two patients were infected through an unknown route of transmission. All of these AIDS patients were farmers in the village. Eight ARV drugs were available for free to these AIDS patients by the national government. Three village doctors from the clinics provided the free ARV counseling services and distributed the ARV drugs. Four of these ARV drugs were manufactured by a number of domestic Chinese pharmaceutical companies, including zidovudine (AZT), didanosine (DDI), stavudine (D4T), and nevirapine (NVP). The other four ARV drugs, including tenofovir (TDF), lamivudine (3TC), efavirenz (EFV), lopinavir and ritonavir (LPV/r), were imported by the Chinese national government.

The author would like to acknowledge the contributions of Yamei Fu, Erhong Zhao, and Ge Zhang of the Wolong Health Center and Deixang Li of the People's Hospital of Shangcai County, Henan Province.

X. Cheng (✉)
Wolong Health Center, Shangcai County, Henan Province, China 463800
e-mail: chxd6933022@163.com

Different ARV Drug Regimens

The majority of these patients (262/271) had been taking ARV drugs for more than 6 months at the beginning of this study. Seven of these patients started their ARV therapies less than 6 months before this study. During the period of this study, approximately 47% of the patients were taking AZT/D4T+3TC+NVP; 26% of them took TDF+3TC+LPV/r; 21% of them took AZT+DDI+NVP, 4% of them took AZT/D4T+3TC+EFV; 1% of them took D4T+DDI+NVP; and 1% of them took D4T+DDI+EFV.

About 30% of these patients had never changed their drug regimens since they started the ARV therapy, whereas 43% of them changed their drug regimens once and 19% of them changed their regimens twice. The remainder of the patients changed their regimens more than twice since they began their ARV therapy.

CD4 Counts and Viral Loads

During the period of this study, the majority of the patients (53%) had their CD4 counts between 200 and 500 (per ml), whereas 29% of the patients had CD4 counts higher than 500 and 18% of them had CD4 counts lower than 200. At the same time, the viral load tests showed that the majority of the patients (58%) had undetectable levels or lower than 400 copies per ml, whereas the ARV therapy failed in nearly 3% of the patients with their viral loads that were higher than 100,000 copies per ml. The other 39% of the patients had viral loads between 400 and 100,000. During the study period, two patients died, and four patients were hospitalized because of AIDS-related severe opportunistic infections.

Compliance

This study measured patient compliance to the ARV therapies. All the patient participants were asked to complete a survey form monthly with help from one of the village clinicians or their DOT (direct observed treatment) monitors, who were either family members or close neighbors with elementary training in the ARV therapy. The survey forms included a daily record of actual drug-taking time. The drug-taking schedule adherence (or schedule compliance) is defined as drugs taken within 2 hour of the morning and evening drug-taking time point. If the total drug-taking schedule compliances were less than 95%, it would be defined as noncompliant. All the patient participants were also asked to save any remaining medication at the end of each month. Then, by calculating the percentage of the remaining medication in the total amount that a patient should have taken, "qualified" drug-taking dose compliances (dose compliance) were defined as the leftover drugs were less than 5%.

The study results showed that 31% of the patients were not qualified as the schedule compliant and 11% of them were not qualified as the dose compliant. Taken together, the total ARV drug noncompliance in this study group was 42%.

Causes of ARV Drug Noncompliance

According to the patient survey results, about half of the schedule noncompliant patients (53%) stated that they simply forgot to take the ARV drugs, whereas 57% of them said that they were too busy with their farm work to take the drugs. However, about 40% of the schedule noncompliant patients blamed the unbearable side effects of the ARV drugs they were taking. In fact, the drug side effects were cited as the main cause for the dose noncompliance as the patients hoped that reducing the drug dosages might make taking the drug more bearable.

Based on some anecdotal reports that the schedule compliances could decrease during the holidays, especially during the most significant holidays for Chinese farmers such as the Spring Festival (Chinese New Year), a special follow-up visit by some of these 271 AIDS patients were conducted after the Spring Festival of 2009. Fifty-two patients were randomly selected to complete a self-reported survey about their ARV drug-taking compliance. To no one's surprise, 69% of the patients chose not to take the ARV drugs on the Chinese New Year's Eve and the following morning.

Coinfections and Liver Disease

Since some of these AIDS patients had started the ARV therapy in 2002, the ALT (alanine aminotransferase) tests were included as part of the clinical tests for this study. Nearly 35% of the patients (94 of 271) had their ATL level higher than 50 U, indicating abnormal liver functions. In fact, four of these AIDS patients had to stop their ARV therapies in order to be first treated for their liver disease.

The liver abnormalities were apparently not all due to the side effects of the ARV drugs. Of these AIDS patients in the group, 113 were also tested for HBV (Hepatitis B virus) and HCV (Hepatitis C) infections. The results showed that 78% of them were co-infected with HCV and nearly 10% of them were tested positive for HBV as well as HCV (triple infections).

Discussion

Previous studies in China showed that at least 95% compliance to the ARV drug-taking schedule and correct dosages would be required to achieve treatment efficacy [1]. The study presented here showcased one of the most basic village treatment units in a rural area of China with a minimum health care infrastructure (a village clinic without any medical equipment) and three village doctors caring for more than 300 AIDS patients, 58% of whom had viral load tests within the treatment-effective scope. However, our study also showed that the noncompliance to the ARV therapies was worrisome (42%), which coincided with the percentage of the ARV treatment failures. Among many medical and nonmedical reasons that caused the ARV therapy noncompliance, some might have been corrected. For example, our survey found that the majority of the patients refused to take their ARV drugs during the Chinese New Year's Eve and the New Year's morning. Some patients even refused to take their medications before the fifth day of the Chinese New Year simply because it was the most important holiday for local farmers. Public education about the fatal consequence of such noncompliance to the ARV therapy is urgently needed.

Severe adverse effects of a long-term ARV therapy, including various side effects of ARV drugs, were the second most significant factor that resulted in the noncompliance to ARV therapy in the rural areas. There were 59 AIDS patients in this study, who began the second-line regimen 1 month before the study started, and who stated that because the side effects of the new regimen were so unbearable, they had to either stop taking the drugs or reduce the amount of the drugs they were supposed to take. Two patients strongly demanded to return to the original first-line therapy, which had failed them.

This study also found that the drug-taking frequency, the dosage, and the type of ARV drugs had significant impact on the patients' compliance. For example, most of the remainder of drugs at the end of each month during this study, which a patient was asked to bring in when given the drugs for the following month by a village doctor, were those pills that should been taken twice a day. It appeared that the more pills per day the patients were told to take, the worse the compliance became. Additionally, all of the patients who had taken the powder form of DDI could not tolerate the taste of the drug. Some patients even felt nauseous when they saw other people handling the DDI powder. The majority of these patients said that they were more likely to take their ARV drugs when the DDI powder could be replaced with the chewable DDI tablets. In fact, after 3TC became available through the National Free ARV Program, many patients noted that 3TC was easier than DDI for them to follow their drug-taking schedule and dosages. It would be advantageous for the patients and doctors alike if newer combinational ARV drugs could become available, thus increasing the ARV compliances. As some of these "ideal" new drugs, which require only one pill a day without significant adverse effects, have been approved by China's State Food and Drug Administration (SFDA) to be sold in China and can be produced by domestic local drug manufacturers as soon as the patents expire in the next decade, it is hopeful that the current ARV therapy efficacy will be improved significantly in the future.

The most worrisome problem in the resource-poor regions like ours was the limited options for the second-line or third-line regimens should an AIDS patient fail his/her first-line regimen. All of our patients depended on the free ARV drugs provided by the national government. As previously mentioned, the free ARV program started with the four drugs made by some domestic Chinese drug manufacturers.

Although four more imported ARV drugs were later included in the program, much more such additions would be required in the near future.

Most of the patients in our clinic, who switched to the second-line ARV regimen, were able to improve their compliance after they were told the dire clinical consequences should they fail to comply again. Despite the increased patient compliance, 17% (12/71) of the patients still chose to reduce their drug dosage or skipped taking their new regimen all together due to the side effects of the drugs. Because of the inability of our local clinic to provide accurate laboratory tests for the appearance of drug-resistant mutant viruses, the choice of the second-line ARV regimen was not based on virology results but only on clinical outcomes or continuous declines of the CD4 counts.

As the AIDS patients in our clinic continued to receive ARV therapies, some of them had started it since 2002, and grew older, an ensuing number of chronic diseases such as hypertension and coronary artery disease, as well as other infections, seemed to appear more frequently. For example, in addition to the aforementioned high rate of HIV-1/HCV coinfection (78%), this study also observed the increasing number of tuberculosis infections in those AIDS patients (9/271). As aforementioned, coinfections like these and other opportunistic infections had resulted in higher noncompliance. Unfortunately, in resource-poor areas, such as ours, we are limited in our ability to overcome these difficulties.

Reference

1. Zhang F (ed) (2008) National free antiretroviral treatment of AIDS manual, 2nd edn. People's Medical Publishing House, Beijing, pp 35, 42, 109–110, 119–123

Chapter 4
HIV/AIDS Treatment and Control in India and the Millennium Development Goals

Srikanth P. Tripathy and Sriram P. Tripathy

Abbreviations

3TC	Lamivudine
AIDS	Acquired immunodeficiency syndrome
ART	Antiretroviral treatment/therapy
ATT	Anti-tuberculosis treatment/therapy
ATV	Atazanavir
CD4 count	CD4 T-lymphocyte count
COE	Centers of excellence
d4T	Stavudine
ddI	Didanosine
EFV	Efavirenz
FTC	Emtricitabine
Hb	Hemoglobin
HIV	Human immunodeficiency virus
IDV	Indinavir
LPV	Lopinavir
NACO	National AIDS Control Organization
NACP	National AIDS Control Program
NNRTI	Non-nucleoside reverse transcriptase inhibitor
NVP	Nevirapine
PI	Protease inhibitor

S.P. Tripathy
National AIDS Research Institute, Pune, India
e-mail: Srikanthtripathy@gmail.com

S.P. Tripathy (✉)
Indian Council of Medical Research, #2 Radhika Vaibhav, Jagtapnagar, Wanawadi,
Pune 411040, India
e-mail: sriramtripathy@hotmail.com

Y. Lu et al. (eds.), *HIV/AIDS Treatment in Resource Poor Countries:*
Public Health Challenges, DOI 10.1007/978-1-4614-4520-3_4,
© Springer Science+Business Media New York 2013

PLHA   People living with HIV/AIDS
RNTCP   Revised National Tuberculosis Control Program
RTV   Ritonavir
SACS   State AIDS Control Society
TB   Tuberculosis disease
TDF   Tenofovir disproxil fumarate
ZDV   Zidovudine

Introduction

Infection with the human immunodeficiency virus (HIV) is unique. It infects only humans and causes mortality in almost every person. The presence of infection goes undetected for years because of lack of symptoms. Progression to HIV-related diseases is slow, taking an average of about 8 years from infection to the development of acquired immunodeficiency syndrome (AIDS), and without specific antiretroviral therapy (ART), the survival period after the appearance of AIDS is 1–2 years. The explosive research undertaken globally during the short span since its recognition in 1981 has provided mankind with the tools to tackle the pandemic effectively with substantial progress made in reducing the transmission of HIV infection, especially from mothers to infants, and in specific treatment with antiretroviral drugs. Today, there is a plethora of drugs available and although no single drug or combination of drugs has so far been found to completely eliminate the virus and affect a cure, many combinations of drugs properly used suppress the multiplication of the virus, ensuring the survival of individual patients for many years and permitting them to lead normal healthy lives until the onset of AIDS.

The Indian Epidemic

India has from the beginning of the global epidemic maintained vigilance against HIV infection. Its efforts in screening risk groups in the early 1980s provided the first evidence of indigenous transmission of HIV in commercial sex workers in Chennai, India, in May 1986 [1]. Since then, efforts have been made continuously to evolve effective control measures initially directed at prevention of infection, reducing the transmission of HIV and the management and care of HIV infected persons, and now fully directed toward successful treatment of patients with ART.

Current Status of the Infection in India

India is a low-income country with a current population of about 1.2 billion. The HIV epidemic level is a concentrated one with substantially higher prevalence among

Table 4.1 HIV prevalence in
India [2]

Category	Estimate
Total population (in 2007)	1.027 billion
HIV prevalence (15–49 years)	
Men	0.40%
Women	0.27%
Both sexes	0.34%
PLHA (adults and children)	2.31 million
Children (below 15 years)	3.8%

Table 4.2 HIV prevalence in
high-risk groups in India
(2007) [3, 4]

Category	Percent positive
ANC attendees	0.48
STD clinic attendees	3.67
IDU	7.23
MSM	7.41
Migrants	3.6
Truckers	2.51

selected high-risk groups (HRGs) than in the general population. Distribution of infection in the country is uneven—in many states, the prevalence is low. In six states—Andhra, Karnataka, Maharashtra, Manipur, Nagaland, and Tamil Nadu— prevalence is high and these states have received greater focus of attention compared to the rest. The country has 609 districts—in 156 districts (Category A), the prevalence of HIV infection in attendees in Antenatal Clinics (ANCs) is over 1%. In an additional 39 districts (Category B), HIV prevalence in ANCs is less than 1% but prevalence in HRGs is over 5%. These 195 districts have received greater attention for the provision of HIV-control measures than the rest of the districts. Based on the HIV sentinel surveillance carried out in 2008–2009, it was estimated that India has about 2.39 million HIV-infected persons with an adult HIV prevalence of about 0.31% [1] (Table 4.1). Nearly all of the people living with AIDS (PLHA) are adults and adolescents. Children comprise only about 3.5% of those infected.

The Most Vulnerable Population and Common Risk Factors

Transmission is largely sexual, and mostly heterosexual with a small proportion due to men having sex with men (MSM). In addition, there is a sizable population of HIV-infected injection drug users (IDUs) in four large cities—Chennai, Mumbai, Delhi, and Chandigarh and in two states in the northeast—Manipur and Nagaland. The rates of prevalence in the categories of HRG and general population (ANC attendees) are indicated in Table 4.2 [3, 4]. These data have been collected through annual HIV sentinel surveillance and represent the findings in 2007 among 358,797 persons tested.

The changes in prevalence in successive years are monitored through annual seroprevalence surveys conducted under the National AIDS Control Program (NACP). It is estimated that there are about 2.5 million men who have sex with men, 0.16 million injecting drug users, and 0.8–1.2 million female sex workers (FSWs) [2].

National Response to the Epidemic and Public Health Measures

The Ministry of Health and Family Welfare has the responsibility for HIV-control activities in India. The program is executed under the guidance of the National AIDS Control Organization (NACO). The apex body has organized three successive National AIDS Control Program: NACP I, II, and III. NACO formulates policies, plans, monitors, executes, coordinates, and evaluates all aspects of AIDS management in India. The current 5-year program, NACP III, was started in 2007. High priority is accorded to measures to promote, prevent, and care, with the objectives of reducing HIV transmission rates, providing care and treatment, and reducing mortality due to AIDS. It has a wide network of government public health entities, including counseling and testing centers, treatment centers, research organizations, and training centers. The management of the program is decentralized with the State AIDS Control Society (SACS) in each state having the responsibility to administer the program and monitor the activities in each district. In addition to the government health facilities in the country, the program is ably assisted and strengthened by outputs from many nongovernmental organizations, WHO, UNAIDS, UNICEF and other international organizations such as the Bill and Melinda Gates Foundation.

Millennium Development Goals and Targets

In 2000, the WHO, the United Nations, and its member countries identified eight developmental goals for socioeconomic development and decreasing disease burden in the world. Goal 6 provided for the combat of HIV/AIDS, malaria, and other diseases, including tuberculosis (TB). For AIDS, the targets were:

– Have halted by 2015 and begun to reverse the spread of HIV/AIDS.
– Achieved by 2010, universal access for treatment for HIV/AIDS for all those who need it.

There is evidence that in India, the epidemic has peaked and is declining slowly [5]. NACP III has set 2011 as the year for halting and reversing the epidemic in India. It is targeted to reduce new infections by 60% in high prevalence states and 40% in vulnerable states.

Table 4.3 National ART regimens in adults and adolescents in India [6, 7]

Regimen	Drugs			Remarks
	NRTI	NNRTI	PI	
Regimen I	AZT+3TC	+NVP		First line/preferred
Regimen Ia	d4T+3TC	+NVP		First line, preferred for patients with Hb <8 g/dl
Regimen II	AZT+3TC	+EFV		First line, preferred for patients on ATT
Regimen IIa	d4T+3TC	+EFV		First line, for patients on ATT and Hb <8 g/dl
Regimen III	TDF+3TC	+NVP		Alternate first line, for patients not tolerating AZT or d4T on NVP-based regimen
Regimen IIIa	TDF+3TC	+EFV		Alternate first line, for patients not tolerating AZT or d4T on EFV-based regimen
Regimen IV	AZT+3TC		LPV/Rit	Second line, for patients not tolerating NVP and EFV
Regimen IVa	d4T+3TC		LPV/Rit	Second line, for patients not tolerating NVP and EFV
Regimen V	AZT+TDF+3TC		LPV/Rit	Second line, preferred for second-line regimen
Regimen Va	TDF+3TC		LPV/Rit	Second line, for patients with anemia <8 g/dl

AZT=zidovudine;   3TC=lamivudine;   EFV=efavirenz;   LPV=lopinavir;   d4T=stavudine; TDF=tenofovir; NVP=nevirapine; Rit=ritonavir

HIV Counseling and Testing

There is a wide network of HIV testing facilities in over 4,000 centers throughout the country. Initially, almost all centers provided client-initiated testing and later, more and more testing centers were provider initiated, related to antenatal care and HRGs. By December 2008, 8.7 million individuals were tested. The coverage was approximately a third of FSWs, IDUs, and MSMs [2].

Antiretroviral Treatment

The advent of antiretroviral treatment (ART) under the "3 by 5" initiative for giving ART to three million PLHA globally by 2005 provided a quantum leap from the largely diagnostic, preventive, and epidemiologic activities under the program to a much higher level of control measures leading to providing access to all PLHA requiring specific ART under a carefully formulated program.

Adults and adolescent PLHA identified as HIV-positive either through client-initiated testing (voluntary testing) or provider-initiated testing facilities, are registered as a pre-ART cohort and monitored periodically, clinically, and by CD4 counts and become eligible for ART when clinically warranted—WHO stage III with a CD4 count below 350 per cubic mm or stage IV, or when the CD4 counts fall below 250 per cubic mm. *All HIV-positive children* are eligible to receive ART. The program has identified a variety of ART regimens [6, 7] (Table 4.3) including combinations of three or four drugs. The combinations of drugs target different stages of the HIV replication cycle, and when used appropriately, they slow down HIV disease progression, reduce the risk of opportunistic infections, and prolong life.

All the drugs are provided free of cost to the patients. Patients collect their supply of drugs once a month either at the ART Centers or at the Link ART Centers (LACs) situated close to the residence of the patient. In December 2010, a total of 387,205 patients [1] including 22,858 children were receiving ART, indicating over 50% increase since December 2008 [8]. The survival rate for patients who have been on treatment for 1 year was about 80%. Response to treatment is monitored through six monthly CD4 counts and if adverse events occurred, they are managed appropriately, including a change of drugs, if necessary.

Treatment Access Sites

In 2010, the program had 292 ART centers, mostly located in urban areas and has a target of adding another 50 centers by the end of NACP III (2011). Patients are registered and initiated into treatment at the *ART Centers*. Thereafter, they can access drugs at the ART Centers or at the LAC located at the patient's residence. Second-line regimens are provided at the ten *Centers of Excellence*.

Prevention, Care, and Management of HIV/TB Co-infection

HIV-related TB poses a serious challenge to the management of HIV. Globally, of 9.27 million incident TB cases, 1.37 million were among the PLHA [9]. About 456,000 PLHA died from TB, constituting about 23% of about two million HIV-related deaths in 2007. India too has to face this challenge, since about 60–70% of the adults in the Indian general population are infected with the tubercle bacillus, with a similar proportion of TB infected among adult HIV-infected persons. TB is a major cause of HIV-related deaths in India—30,000 TB patients with HIV died in 2007, and the prevalence of HIV in incident cases of TB was 5.3%. The management of HIV–TB co-infection has therefore been accorded very high priority. Both the national programs in India, Revised National TB Control Program (RNTCP) and the NACP, are well formulated and are effectively implemented and indeed, each of the programs is a model for the other countries to emulate. Close coordination exists between the two programs.

Cohorts of PLHA are subjected to intensive TB case finding. TB cases detected among the PLHA are registered under the RNTCP, and are treated with standard anti-tuberculosis (ATT) regimens under the directly observed therapy short course (DOTS) strategy. The TB cure rate among patients without HIV is over 90% under RNTCP. Success rates in TB patients with HIV are however lower, since 20–30% of HIV–TB patients die during ATT therapy. The intensified TB case-finding activity among PLHA results in the detection and treatment of TB in early stages, however, patients initially diagnosed as TB under the RNTCP and subsequently identified as co-infected with HIV through provider-related HIV testing usually have advanced TB disease with high levels of immunosuppression, and 20–30% of them die in early months of treatment. Current policy is to initiate ART in TB patients soon after initiation of ATT, ensuring the availability of the benefits of immune recovery to the HIV/TB patient, with possible reduction in HIV-related mortality.

Management of TB under RNTCP

All newly diagnosed, previously untreated cases of TB are treated with a standard 6-month regimen (Category I) consisting of four drugs—ethambutol, isoniazid, rifampicin, and pyrazinamide—EHRZ—given three times a week for 2 months followed by treatment with rifampicin and isoniazid three times a week for another period of 4 months. This regimen is highly effective and cure rates of over 90% have been achieved under the RNTCP. TB patients who had failed on other drug regimens and are still having active disease, and those who fail on the Category I regimen are treated with a 8-month retreatment regimen—Category II—consisting of 2 months of treatment with five drugs—EHRZ supplemented with streptomycin -S- for 2 months, followed by EHRZ for another month, and a successive 5 months of EHR, all administered thrice weekly. This regimen is also highly effective for TB with success rates of about 70%. Thus, only a few remaining patients who have failed on Category I and II regimens, need to be treated under a DOTS—Plus Strategy with regimens comprising of five or six drugs capable of overcoming multi-drug resistant TB, which is likely to emerge in a few cases in the event of failure of Category II regimen [10].

Management of TB in HIV/TB Patients

The management of TB in HIV/TB patients is similar to the management in those who are not HIV-infected [11, 12]. The ATT drug regimens are equally effective in both categories of patients with one exception. In some HIV/TB patients, diagnosis of TB might have been delayed and the mortality rates during treatment are likely to be higher with some mortality due to advanced TB and some due to HIV-related causes. Close coordination and interaction between the RNTCP and the NACP ensures that HIV/TB patients started on ATT are assessed concurrently for ART and are initiated in ART within weeks of commencing ATT. Successful TB treatment and improvement in immunocompetency following ART initiation ensures reduction in morbidity and mortality.

Immune Reconstitution Inflammatory Syndrome

During the treatment of HIV/TB patients with ATT as well as ART regimens, there is a risk of the occurrence of an episode of IRIS—immune reconstitution inflammatory

Table 4.4 Prevention of mother-to-child transmission through ART Jan–Dec 2008 [14]

Category	Number	Coverage
Pregnant women tested	4,234,401	16%
Estimated pregnant women with HIV	49,000	–
Pregnant women on ART for PMTCT	10,673	22%
Infants born to HIV + women receiving ART for PMTCT	10,577	22%

syndrome—occurring in 10–30% of cases on ATT and ART within weeks of initiating ART [13]. It occurs mostly in HIV/TB patients who have low CD4 cell counts at the time of initiation of ATT, and the sudden improvement in the immunocompetence following initiation of ART results in adverse inflammatory events in TB. In a typical case, a TB patient who is on ATT and is showing a favorable response to ATT is started on ART. Within weeks of initiation of ART, paradoxically there is sudden deterioration in TB with manifestation of fever, clinical or radiographic worsening of the TB lesions, and/or appearance of TB lesions in new sites. Most of these IRIS events are of short duration and are easily managed with steroids or anti-inflammatory agents without interruption of ATT or ART. Occasionally, the reactions are severe and cause fatality. TB/HIV patients receiving ATT and ART have to be monitored for possible occurrence of IRIS, which should be attended to as soon as symptoms of IRIS become manifest.

Prevention of Mother-to-Child Transmission

By 2008, as many as 4,817 health facilities were providing prevention of mother-to-child transmission (PMTCT) services including testing of pregnant women for HIV and provision of antiretroviral prevention such as single dose of nevirapine to mothers at the time of delivery and testing and follow up of infants born to HIV-positive mothers. By December 2009, about 16% of 27 million total annual pregnancies were covered under the PMTCT: 10,673 HIV-positive pregnant women received nevirapine for PMTCT [14] (Table 4.4). CD4 counts were done on 1,033 pregnant women. While 325 of them were found eligible for ART, 220 (68%) actually started on ART. It is estimated that 63,889 children were living with HIV, with perinatal transmission being the major source of infection. Currently, 22,858 of children living with AIDS are receiving ART. There is a plan to steadily scale up the PTMCT over the years under NACP IV (2012–2016) and it is expected that by 2016, about 48,000 HIV-positive pregnant women will be identified and provided PTMCT.

Management of Other Opportunistic Infections

The program has close links with general health systems and appropriate referral arrangements. PLHA developing events of HIV-associated opportunistic infections are referred to medical college hospitals and other health facilities for appropriate management including identification of the infecting organisms and their management. Apart from TB, the most common opportunistic infections encountered in India are candidial infections, toxoplasmosis, and cryptococcal infections.

Malignancies such as Kaposi's sarcoma are not commonly seen in HIV-infected patients in India. The provision of health care free of charge to PLHA, making the diagnostic and treatment facilities available through a wide network of facilities provides hope of survival to a large body of PLHA. Hope for survival is the driving force, which calls for and ensures a level of lifelong adherence to ART, which would have been inconceivable for any other disease.

Adherence/Retention of Patients on ART

Treatment is lifelong and the drugs need to be taken daily, some once a day and others twice a day. Experience in the management of ATT (without HIV) has taught us that even in regimens of 6 months duration, some slippage in compliance during the later months of treatment do occur. For lifelong ART regimens, the challenge of maintaining high levels of adherence to treatment, and especially so in the later months—24, 36, 48 months onward, has to be met with continuous monitoring, keeping track of drug collections, timely detection of defaulters and prompt retrieval measures, and periodic examination of the CD4 levels. Some of the large ART centers in India have achieved adherence levels of over 90% as assessed at 12 months of ART. There is some decline thereafter, partly because of migration out of the area and death in some cases, but the percentage of patients available for follow up is still large. Many patients have survived for over 5 years with ART and are leading a productive and otherwise healthy life. The credit for the success of the program goes to the entire team of workers in the NACO and the NACP participants and to the many nongovernmental organizations, private practitioners, WHO, UNAIDS, UNICEF, and other international organizations such as the Bill and Melinda Gates Foundation.

Other Preventive Interventions

A dual epidemic of transmission among IDUs and sexual transmission is present in two northeastern states of Manipur and Nagaland [15]. In addition, transmission of HIV among IDUs in large cities like Chennai, Mumbai, and Delhi is also contributing to the HIV burden in India. PLHA in these HRGs have access to the ART services. For all IDUs, harm reduction interventions are delivered through 323 needle–syringe program sites and 46 opioid substitution therapy sites where buprenorphine is provided to IDUs as substitution therapy. STI services are provided at 245 targeted intervention sites [8]. The coverage of IDUs, FSWs, and MSMs by preventive services in 2008 was 40–45%.

Future Risks and Worst-Case Scenarios

There is evidence from annual sentinel surveillance data that the epidemic in India has peaked [5]. With the implementation of prevention and treatment programs under the NACP, it is hoped that transmission rates will continue to decline in future years and life expectancy in PLHA will go up substantially. However, this presupposes that the present tempo of effectiveness will be continued and scaled up, calling for substantial investment in men, material, and money. The world has seen an economic slowdown recently, but India has so far managed to avert any financial crisis. There is substantial commitment to both AIDS Control and TB Control programs. ART and ATT drugs are available at reasonable prices for the programs. Should the international economic situation worsen and assistance is scaled down, there may be a resultant downturn in some activities of the Control Programs; this, however, is unlikely to affect the goals and achievements of the NACP III. The budgetary requirement of about $2.5 billion for NACP III has been provided largely through domestic funding, and by funding from donor agencies [2]. A mid-term review of the NACP III conducted in December 2009 [16] has revealed that the program is well on its track and the findings provide material for the planning of NACP IV commencing in 2012. It is expected that NACP IV (2012–2016) will provide further up-scaling of the activities, including greater coverage of ART in PLHA and large-scale support for research activities related to program assistance and evaluation. Universal access to ART by 2015 by all PLHA needing treatment, as envisaged by the Millennium Development Goal, would be well within sight. However, the proposed changes in the eligibility criteria for treatment, making people eligible for ART initiation in earlier stages would require much larger coverage than the target under current eligibility criteria and may delay the achievement of the target beyond 2015.

Urgent Needs and Action Steps

There are about 292 ART centers spread over different parts of the country, the majority of them in states with high HIV prevalence. The network needs to be further widened to reach the remote rural areas, to ensure access to treatment is available in all parts of India. The programs for the prevention of transmission of HIV from mother to child need to be carefully monitored to ensure larger coverage, monitoring emergence of drug resistance in the mother and in the infected babies.

Many research activities have been undertaken in India, especially in areas of epidemiology and PMTCT. There is a need to step up research activities in chemotherapy—for formulation of better regimens, monitoring drug resistance related to ART, and newer approaches to treatment such as the recently proposed test-and-treat policy where all persons who are diagnosed as HIV positive become eligible for treatment.

While challenges appear to be formidable, data show that the program is functioning effectively, as reflected in a decline in the prevalence rates over the years from 0.45% in 2002 till 0.34% in 2008. Five of the six high prevalence states which had a rate over 1% in ANC Clinic attendees, now have a prevalence of less than 1%. The NACP policies are sound and practical and hold great promise. The policies and programs are constantly evolving and changing with innovation and improvisation as the program continues. Target 6a of the Millennium Goal for HIV aims to have halted by 2015 and begun to reverse the spread of HIV–AIDS and this target is very likely to be met in India. Target 6b provides for achievement by 2010 universal access to treatment for HIV/AIDS to all who need them. With a sound NACP, political commitment, and committed health care and research personnel, India is well poised to meet both the millennium goals.

References

1. National AIDS Control Organization (2010) Annual report 2010–2011. Government of India, NACO, Department of AIDS Control, Ministry of Health and Family Welfare
2. World Health Organization Regional Office for South East Asia (2009) HIV/AIDS in the South-East Asia region, 2009
3. National AIDS Control Organization (2006) Report of the Expert Group on the estimation of populations with high risk behavior for NACP III Planning; The National AIDS Control Program Phase III (2006–2011). Ministry of Health and Family Welfare, India, 2006
4. National AIDS Control Organization (2007) Annual HIV sentinel survey—country report
5. Simoes EA, Babu PG, John TJ, Nirmala S, Solomon S, Lakshminarayana CS et al (1987) Evidence for HTLV-III infection in prostitutes in Tamil Nadu (India). Indian J Med Res 85:335–338
6. National AIDS Control Organization (2008) NACO guidelines on second line ART for adults and adolescents. In: Meeting of technical research group, 28–29 Aug 2009
7. National AIDS Control Organization (2010) National guidelines in second line ART for adults and adolescents (Draft 2010). National AIDS Control Organization
8. World Health Organization (2009) Towards universal access. Scaling up priority HIV/AIDS intimation in the health sector—program report 2009. World Health Organization, Geneva, http://www.who.int/hiv/pub/2009progressreport/en/index.html. Accessed 10 Apr 2010
9. World Health Organization (2009) Global tuberculosis control 2009: epidemiology, strategy, financing. WHO report 2009. WHO/HTM/TB/2009.411
10. Chauhan LS (2008) Drug resistant TB: RNTCP response. Indian J Tuberculosis 55:5–8
11. World Health Organization (2009) Global tuberculosis control. A short update to the 2009 report. WHO, Geneva, WHO/HTM/TB/2009.426
12. World Health Organization (2009) Global tuberculosis control 2009: epidemiology, strategy, planning. World Health Organization, Geneva
13. Meintjes G, Lawn SD, Scano F et al (2008) Tuberculosis associated immune resonstitution syndrome: case definitions for use in resource limited settings. Lancer Infect Dis 8:516, Personal view (http://www.thelancet.com/infection)
14. World Health Organization (2005) WHO and UNAIDS. Progress on global access to HIV antiretroviral therapy: an update on '3 by 5'. World Health Organization, Geneva, http://www.who.int/3by5/publications/progressreport/en. Accessed 18 Apr 2010
15. Mahanta J, Medhi GK, Paranjape RS, Roy N, Kohli A, Akoijam B et al (2008) Injecting and sexual risk behaviour, sexually transmitted infections and HIV prevalence in injecting drug users in three states in India. AIDS 22(suppl 5):S59–S68

16. National AIDS Control Organization (2010) NACO News—a newsletter of the National AIDS Control Organization 4(8)
17. UNAIDS (2009) AIDS epidemic update: Nov 2009. UNAIDS/09.36E/JC 1700 E:1–100
18. UNAIDS, WHO (2009) AIDS epidemic update. World Health Organization, Geneva
19. United Nations (2001) United Nations millennium development goals. United Nations, New York, http://www.un.org/milleniumgoals

Chapter 5
HIV Treatment Scale-up in Africa: The Impact of Drug Resistance

Nzovu Ulenga and Phyllis J. Kanki

Introduction

The HIV/AIDS pandemic has evolved into one of the greatest global public health challenges in recent history. It has progressed unchecked in many parts of the world for close to three decades. An estimated 1.8 million people were newly infected with HIV in sub-Saharan Africa in 2009, while 22.5 million people were estimated to be living with HIV. Globally, 33.3 million people are living with HIV, and ~22 million reside in Africa, and 1.3 of the 1.8 million AIDS deaths in 2009 are estimated in sub-Saharan Africa [1]. In this region, the HIV epidemics vary significantly from country to country, in both scale and scope. Adult national HIV prevalence is below 2% in several countries of West and Central Africa, as well as in the horn of Africa, but as early as 2007 it exceeded 15% in Southern African countries, and was above 5% in Central and East Africa (Fig. 5.1) [2].

In recent times, due to prevention and treatment efforts, HIV prevalence rates have seemed to stabilize, although at very high levels, particularly in southern Africa, whose ten countries bear one-third of the HIV epidemic on the continent. In a growing number of countries, adult HIV prevalence rates are falling. In Zimbabwe, HIV prevalence in adults fell from 26% in 2002 to 15.3% in 2007. In Botswana, HIV prevalence among adults dropped from 26.5% in 2001 to 17.6% in 2008 [3]. HIV data from antenatal clinics in South Africa suggest that the country's epidemic might be stabilizing as well. The estimated 5.6 million South Africans living with HIV in 2009 make this the largest HIV epidemic in the world [1]. Meanwhile, the 26% HIV prevalence found in adults in Swaziland in 2009 is the highest prevalence ever documented in a national population-based survey anywhere in the world [1].

N. Ulenga • P.J. Kanki (✉)
Department of Immunology and Infectious Diseases, Harvard School of Public Health,
651 Huntington Avenue, Boston, MA 02115, USA
e-mail: nulenga@hsph.harvard.edu; pkanki@hsph.harvard.edu

Y. Lu et al. (eds.), *HIV/AIDS Treatment in Resource Poor Countries:*
Public Health Challenges, DOI 10.1007/978-1-4614-4520-3_5,
© Springer Science+Business Media New York 2013

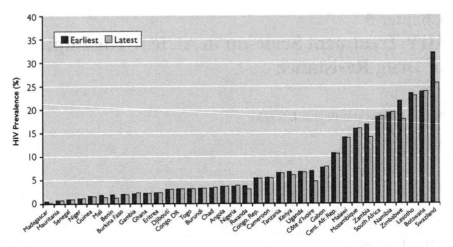

Fig. 5.1 HIV prevalence rate among adults aged 15–49 for 2003–2007. Source: UNAIDS 2006 and 2007 reports on the global AIDS epidemic

In East Africa, HIV prevalence has either reached a plateau or is decreasing and adult national HIV prevalence in Uganda has stabilized between 6 and 7% [3]. HIV epidemics in West Africa are stable or are declining, as is the case for Burkina Faso, Ivory Coast, and Mali. In Ivory Coast, HIV prevalence among pregnant women in urban areas fell from 10% in 2001 to 6.9% in 2005. The largest epidemic in West Africa is in Nigeria; the continent's most populous country appears to have stabilized at 3.6%. Despite a relatively low HIV prevalence, Nigeria has the second highest HIV disease burden in the world due to its population size of over 150 million [4, 5].

HIV Treatment in Africa

In 2001, the United Nations endorsed the Declaration of Commitment on HIV/AIDS that recognized that care, support, and treatment of HIV are fundamental elements of an effective response to HIV/AIDS problem. In July 2002, the World Health Organization (WHO) and UNAIDS unveiled the "3 by 5" initiative, with a goal of placing three million people in developing countries on antiretroviral drugs by the end of 2005. Africa responded to UN and WHO initiatives by establishing comprehensive programs to address the HIV/AIDS epidemic.

In March 2001, Festus Mogae, the President of Botswana, announced that his government hoped to implement a national treatment program before the end of the year. This was one of the first times an African country had proposed such an ambitious program. The aim was to provide treatment to 19,000 people. As a result of limited resources, it was decided that the program would initially target four population groups: pregnant women with AIDS, HIV-infected pediatric in-patients, people coinfected with HIV and tuberculosis, and adult patients hospitalized with AIDS.

The Botswana National Antiretroviral Therapy Program was given the name MASA, the Setswana word for "dawn," and the first antiretroviral drugs were provided at the Princess Marina Hospital in Gaborone in January 2002. By May 2004, more than 24,000 people had been enrolled in MASA, of whom 14,000 were receiving antiretroviral treatment (ART). By the end of the year, it was estimated that between 36,000 and 39,000 people were receiving ART, including those accessing ART through the private sector, about a quarter of the total. MASA was achieving good rates of treatment adherence in terms of self-reporting, pill counts, and attending scheduled appointments, and this was confirmed by high rates of viral load suppression. By June 2005, 43,000 people were receiving ART, more than half of the 75,000 in need. According to WHO's figures, 85% of people in need of the drugs were receiving them at the end of the year, including those using the private sector. Number of people receiving ART increased further to 170,000 in 2010, averting an estimated 50,000 AIDS-related deaths [1].

In 2000, the Government of Nigeria started an ambitious ART program with the aim of supplying 10,000 adults and 5,000 children with antiretroviral drugs within 1 year [4]. An initial $3.5 million worth of generic ARVs were to be imported from India and delivered at a subsidized monthly cost of $7 per person. The PEPFAR (United States President's Emergency Plan For AIDS Relief)-supported ART program began in 2004, and by 2006, 41 AIDS treatment centers were providing free ARVs to eligible AIDS patients. Due to increases in HIV/AIDS funding as a result of donations from the Global Fund, PEPFAR, Clinton Foundation, and World Bank, treatment scale-up between 2006 and 2007 was impressive, the number of individuals receiving ARVs increased from 81,000 to 198,000 by the end of 2007, and over 400,000 in 2011.

In 2003, the William J Clinton Foundation and a group of Tanzanian experts created a step-by-step Care and Treatment Plan (2003–2008), which was then adopted by the Tanzanian cabinet. By 2004, only about 0.5% of those with advanced HIV infection and AIDS were receiving the necessary ART. A total of $539 million for a 5-year period was committed to rolling out the AIDS treatment program, with the majority of funds coming from PEPFAR or USAID/PEPFAR and the Global Fund. The Tanzanian government spending on antiretroviral drugs increased from $2 million in 2003 to $17 million in 2005. In March 2009, about 235,000 people with advanced HIV infection had been enrolled, out of the estimated 440,000 in need of care and ART [6].

Treatment Guidelines

To accelerate the scaling up of ART delivery in resource-limited countries, the WHO developed treatment protocols based on simplified guidelines and a decentralized service delivery [7, 8]. Inadequate numbers of trained physicians, nurses, and other healthcare providers and the need for extensive laboratory monitoring of patients required this simplification in many settings in Africa. The WHO protocol enabled healthcare workers with basic training to treat a large numbers of patients. Clinical decision making was largely guided by clinical observation, WHO clinical staging, hematology, biochemistry values, and CD4+ T-cell counts, when available. Originally the standard first-line regimen consisted of two nucleoside reverse transcriptase inhibitors (NRTIs) (3TC and either ZDV or d4T) plus a non-nucleoside reverse transcriptase inhibitor (NNRTI) (either nevirapine (NVP) or efavirenz (EFV)) or a triple NRTI regimen. Regimens using the tenofovir-based NRTI (TDF+3TC (or FTC)+EFV/NVP) were often recommended for patients with HIV/HBV coinfection, but the higher cost of these regimens were an individual country guideline consideration. In 2010, WHO revised their ART guidelines and recommend the use of tenofovir as first-line regimens. Second-line regimens normally consisted of a boosted protease inhibitor (PI) with at least one NRTI [9]. ZDV and d4T are thymidine analog drugs and both select for a common set of mutations called thymidine analog mutations (TAMs). Accumulated TAMs induce cross-resistance to other NRTIs. Both 3TC and NNRTIs have a low genetic barrier to resistance development, thus making the current standard first-line therapies vulnerable to resistance. Due to high costs of PIs in Africa, their use has been limited to second-line therapy use. Given that fewer regimens options are available in most ART programs in Africa, drug resistance is predicted to increase from its current levels in Africa.

HIV Drug Resistance

Access to ART for eligible patients in many African countries has greatly improved over the past few years. However, data on long-term clinical outcomes of individuals receiving ART, the prevalence and patterns of HIV resistance to antiretroviral drugs, and implications of subtype diversity in resistance remains limited. In the rest of this chapter we explore the available data on HIV-1 resistance to antiretroviral drugs in Africa, in relation to the drug regimens used, HIV-1 subtype diversity, and the prevalence of transmitted resistance. We examine data on HIV resistance associated with treatment, prevention of mother-to-child transmission, and transmitted resistance.

The Development of HIV Drug Resistance

The HIV-1 replication process is error-prone, leading to a high rate of mutations [10, 11]. Given the rapid viral turnover [12, 13], accumulation of genetically distinct viruses called quasispecies in an infected individual occur readily. The diversity of the quasispecies changes over the course of infection in response to the host immune response, as well as the use of antiretroviral drugs. Drug resistance occurs upon incomplete suppression of viral replication when optimal drug levels are not maintained, either through non-adherence, treatment interruptions, or the use of suboptimal drug regimens. Drug resistance can also be a result of transmission of a resistant virus to a newly infected individual. Each antiretroviral drug has its own resistance mutations profile, which could be specific to the drug or a class of drugs [14]. Drugs with a high genetic barrier, such as PIs, require the accumulation of more than one mutation to overcome antiviral drug activity. On the other hand, drugs with a low genetic barrier, including lamivudine and NNRTIs, only require a single-point mutation to confer resistance.

Factors That Influence the Development of HIV-1 Drug Resistance in Africa

In Africa, poorly developed health systems create the conditions for the development of drug resistance in patients. There is insufficient laboratory capacity and financial resources to perform the optimal, regular virological monitoring in patients on ART. In the absence of virologic monitoring, ART is primarily monitored by clinical and immunological parameters alone. The low sensitivity and specificity of these latter methods leads to unnecessary switches to second-line ART in the absence of virological failure, and increasing the risk that patients remain on a failing regimen for longer periods [15], which may result in further accumulation of resistance mutations. The availability of adequate second-line drug combinations is also limited in most African settings, such that patients failing first-line therapy may not have sufficient choices for second-line therapy further promoting the development of drug resistance. Additionally, there are important social and environmental factors that pose barriers to the ability of patients to adhere to the complexities of ART. These include the cost and logistics of regular transportation to the clinic for drug pickups and regular clinic visits, the necessity of food, infection control and prophylaxis, and access to services represent challenges to the overall efficacy of ART implementation.

The complexities of regular supply chains for ART drugs and monitoring laboratory tests also represent challenges to the African healthcare systems already burdened by poor regulation, deficiencies in the training of the healthcare workforce, and inadequate healthcare facilities that are regularly maintained [16, 17]. Moreover, Africa is facing shortages of nurses and doctors [18], and these problems ultimately affect the quality of care, which are important factors in prevention of drug resistance. In the early ART treatment programs in Africa, reliance on ART drugs based on low cost often resulted in the use of drugs with low genetic barriers to resistance and high levels of toxicity. In the future, the long-term side effects of some of those frequently used drugs, such as d4T, could negatively affect adherence, thus promoting resistance. Finally, concomitant use of particular tuberculosis drugs such as rifampin could affect the blood levels of antiretroviral drugs such as PIs and EFV, and requires the replacement with rifabutin in order to effectively treat both diseases [19]. This is especially important because of high rates of tuberculosis coinfection in Africa.

HIV-1 Subtype Diversity and Drug Resistance

HIV-1 can be divided into three groups that are genetically distinct: M, N, and O. Groups N and O represent a small minority of HIV-1 infections in central Africa [20, 21], group M is responsible for over 90% of HIV-1 infections globally, and has nine subtypes A–D, F–H, J, and K, and circulating recombinant forms (CRFs) [22, 23]. Subtype C is responsible for 56% of infections in Africa, mainly in Southern and Eastern Horn regions. Smaller proportions of infections are caused by subtypes A (14%), G (10%), CRF02_AG (7%), and other recombinants (9%) mainly in West Africa [24]. Subtype B predominates in Europe, North America, and Australia. Published data suggests that in the first 6–12 months of therapy there is no difference between patients in Africa and patients in developed countries in terms of immunological and virologic outcomes on ART [25–27].

DNA sequences of drug-naive virus isolates of non-B subtypes have shown that 53% and 48% of protease (PR) and reverse transcriptase (RT) positions, respectively, are naturally polymorphic, as compared to subtype B [28, 29]. In subtype B, some polymorphisms at specific amino acid residues such as PR positions 10, 20, 36, 63, 71, 77, and 93; RT positions 69, 75, 98, 106, 118, 179, and 214 are known to be associated with resistance [28, 29]. The extent to which the abundance of polymorphisms in the non-B subtypes alters drug susceptibility or clinical response to therapy is not entirely clear. Polymorphisms such as the frequently occurring M36I in PR, could restore or support the replication capacity of resistant virus hence facilitating the emergence of resistance under drug pressure [30, 31].

Interestingly, there is no current evidence that non-B subtypes viruses develop resistance by mutations at positions that have not been associated with resistance in subtype B viruses [28]. Analysis of various subtypes concluded that the overall genetic barrier to resistance was similar across HIV-1 subtypes [32]. Also, resistance data from Nigeria indicate that drug resistance mutation patterns are similar across subtypes for the most prevalent mutations such as the NRTI mutations M184V/I, T215Y/F and the NNRTI mutations Y181C/I, K103N, and G190A/S. However, subtype-specific differences were found in the M41L and D67N TAMs mutations and the V90I and A98G mutations associated with etravirine resistance [30, 33] (Fig. 5.2a, b). In vitro studies have shown that TDF drug might select the K65R mutation more rapidly in subtype C than in subtype B [34]. Similarly, EFV rapidly selected for the V106M mutation in subtype C, as opposed to the Y181C mutation in subtype B [35]. This could be explained by a subtype difference in the genetic barrier to resistance: the wild-type V106A needs two nucleotide changes in subtype B, as opposed to one in subtype C. Moreover, several studies have demonstrated subtype differences in frequency and long-term persistence of resistance mutations in women and infants after the use of SD-NVP for perinatal mother-to-child transmission (PMTCT) [36].

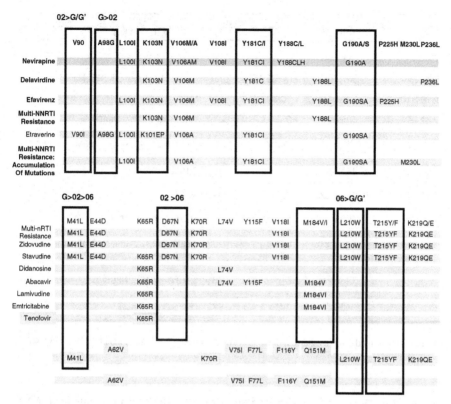

Fig. 5.2 (**a**) Drug resistance mutations associated with NNRTIs by subtypes in Nigerians patients participating in Harvard PEPFAR treatment program. No significant subtypes based differences were observed in pattern and profile of mutations among patients for K103N, Y181C/I and G190A/S. Subtype CRF02_A/G was likely to have V90I mutations compared with subtypes G and G', and subtype G was more like to have A98G mutation than CRF02_A/G. (**b**) Drug resistance mutations associated with NRTIs by subtypes in Nigerians patients participating in Harvard PEPFAR treatment program. No significant subtypes based differences were observed in pattern and profile of mutations among patients

Drug Resistance Among Patients on ART

Observational data from patients on a first-line ART regimens in Africa show large variations in the rate of resistance, reported at 3.7–49% after at least 24 weeks on therapy [34], and the most common mutations are M184V, K103N, and Y181C. In Ivory Coast, South Africa, Uganda, Malawi, and Zimbabwe, the most common PMTCT-associated mutations detected were K103N and Y181C. Resistance rates

Study year	Country	Subtype	N	Mutations
2001	South Africa	C	56	G190A, K103N, A98G
2001	Botswana	C	71	None
2001-2002	Ivory Coast	CRF02_AG	107	K101E, K103N, P236L, K219Q, N88D
2000-20002	Cameroon	CCRF02_AG	128	None
2002	Djibouti	C	47	L100I, K65R, PR: N88D
2002	DRC	Multiple	70	K103N, V179D, M46L, L90M
2002	Burundi	C	101	G190E
2003	Mozambique	C	58	None
2003	Burkina Faso	CRF02_AG	97	M41L, T69S, L33F
2001-2004	Cameroon	CFR02_AG	102	A62V, T69N, V108I, M184V, P236L
2001-2004	Cameroon	CRF02_AG	96	L210W, T215S, N88S
2005-2006	Tanzania	A, C	39	None

Fig. 5.3 Transmitted drug resistance mutations in Africa between 2001 and 2006 [4, 9, 20, 28, 32, 40]

ranged from 19% to 69% in women and from 40% to 87% in infants [36]. NVP resistance at 4–8 weeks postpartum was estimated at 52.6% in infants receiving SD-NVP only at delivery and 16.5% in infants with additional postpartum antiretroviral drugs [37].

Excluding PMTCT-associated resistance, the reported resistance rates, in general, do not appear to exceed rates reported in industrialized countries, where the prevalence of resistance mutations has been estimated at 9% in patients after 2 years on ART, rising to 27% by 6 years [38]. Resistance outcome data on second-line regimens in Africa remains limited [39]. Even less is known about the rate of resistance in children on ART. Studies have reported rates of resistance among treatment-naive individuals in Africa [9, 40–44] (Fig. 5.3). NNRTI resistance rates ranged from 0% to 5.6%, NRTI resistance ranged from 0% to 3.7% and primary PI mutations were rare. Thus, transmitted drug resistance in Africa appears to be relatively low compared to industrialized countries where it is estimated between 9% and 20% [45, 46]. However, the studies from African settings have small sample sizes and differ in assay methodology, the time period in which data were collected, and the population under study. Therefore, there is a need to bolster efforts in surveying the rates and characteristics of transmitted drug resistance in Africa, as the scale-up of ART programs in recent times may increase the risks for transmitted resistance and have a significant impact on the efficacy and implementation of the current ART programs.

The Way Forward: Public Health and Research Priorities

As the number of patients on ART in Africa grows, specific measures are needed to maintain the momentum in the rollout of treatment and prevention programs, while developing effective strategies to control and prevent drug resistance. The limited availability of virological monitoring, detection of resistance mutations, and availability of second- and third-line therapies, poses significant challenges to the long-term efficacy of these programs. Research to determine the ART regimens with prolonged clinical efficacy are urgently needed, and adherence to therapy must be promoted by finding new ways to help patients overcome barriers to adherence in resource-limited settings. In addition, research is needed to determine alternative methods to inform switching from first-line to second-line therapy, in the absence of virologic monitoring.

Laboratory capacity in Africa should be improved to fully accommodate patient monitoring in areas such as hematology, biochemistry, CD4+ T-cell counts, and viral load testing. Currently, the use of conventional resistance detection methods such as genotypic and phenotypic assays, are limited by costs, high capital investment, and the technically skilled staff required to perform these assays. At present, WHO does not recommend resistance testing for individual patient management in resource-limited settings, although this is recommended in developed countries. The development of affordable and more practical alternatives for laboratory monitoring tools, including resistance assays, simple specimen carrier devices, in-house genotyping protocols, and single nucleotide mutation assays such as the ligation amplification assay, should be pursued actively.

Currently, in Africa, the emergence of acquired and transmitted resistance is not routinely evaluated as part of treatment programs. There is a need to determine the proportion of HIV-infected individuals who have developed resistance mutations, and the patterns of such mutations. In addition, the elucidation of specific factors associated with resistance emergence and spread will provide crucial information for adjusting national and international treatment guidelines accordingly. The initiation and significant roll-out of ART programs in Africa has already demonstrated a significant impact on the epidemiology of the epidemic. In order to further support the successful roll-out of these programs and to ensure the sustainability of the achieved quality of care, the importance of drug resistance testing to inform both clinical and public health policies should be considered and implemented in future health system strengthening efforts.

References

1. UNAIDS (2010) Botswana: progress towards universal access and the declaration of commitment on HIV/AIDS. UNAIDS, Geneva
2. UNAIDS (2010) AIDS epidemic update. http://data.unaids.org/pub/Report/2009/JCI700EpiUpdate2009en.pdf

3. UNAIDS/WHO (2008) Epidemiological fact sheets on HIV and AIDS, 2008 updates. UNAIDS, Geneva
4. Kanki P (2009) The challenge and response in Nigeria. In: Kanki P, Marlink R (eds) A line drawn in the sand: responses to the AIDS treatment crisis in Africa. Harvard Center for Population and Development Studies, Cambridge, MA, pp 63–91
5. USAID (2008) Africa region: HIV/AIDS health profile. USAID
6. TACAID (2008) Tanzania: Country progress report. UNAIDS, Geneva
7. Gilks CF, Crowley S, Ekpini R, Gove S, Perriens J, Souteyrand Y et al (2006) The WHO public-health approach to antiretroviral treatment against HIV in resource-limited settings. Lancet 368:505–510
8. WHO (2006) Antiviral therapy for HIV infection in adults and adolescents: recommendations for public health approach. World Health Organization, Geneva
9. WHO (2010) Antiretroviral therapy for HIV infection in adults and adolescents, recommendations for a public health approach
10. Preston BD (1997) Reverse transcriptase fidelity and HIV-1 variation. Science 275:228–229, author reply 230–221
11. Roberts JD, Bebenek K, Kunkel TA (1988) The accuracy of reverse transcriptase from HIV-1. Science 242:1171–1173
12. Ho DD, Neumann AU, Perelson AS, Chen W, Leonard JM, Markowitz M (1995) Rapid turnover of plasma virions and CD4 lymphocytes in HIV-1 infection. Nature 373:123–126
13. Wei X, Ghosh SK, Taylor ME, Johnson VA, Emini EA, Deutsch P et al (1995) Viral dynamics in human immunodeficiency virus type 1 infection. Nature 373:117–122
14. Johnson VA, Brun-Vezinet F, Clotet B, Gunthard HF, Kuritzkes DR, Pillay D et al (2007) Update of the drug resistance mutations in HIV-1: 2007. Top HIV Med 15:119–125
15. Bisson GP, Frank I, Gross R, Lo Re V 3rd, Strom JB, Wang X et al (2006) Out-of-pocket costs of HAART limit HIV treatment responses in Botswana's private sector. AIDS 20:1333–1336
16. Cohen GM (2007) Access to diagnostics in support of HIV/AIDS and tuberculosis treatment in developing countries. AIDS 21(suppl 4):S81–S87
17. Nugent R, Pickett J, Back E (2008) Drug resistance as global health policy priority. Center for Global Development, Washington, DC
18. WHO (2006) The World Health report, 2006. World Health Organization, Geneva
19. Breen RA, Swaden L, Ballinger J, Lipman MC (2006) Tuberculosis and HIV co-infection: a practical therapeutic approach. Drugs 66:2299–2308
20. Fonjungo PN, Dash BC, Mpoudi EN, Torimiro JN, Alemnji GA, Eno LT et al (2000) Molecular screening for HIV-1 group N and simian immunodeficiency virus cpz-like virus infections in Cameroon. AIDS 14:750–752
21. Jaffe HW, Schochetman G (1998) Group O human immunodeficiency virus-1 infections. Infect Dis Clin North Am 12:39–46
22. Grobler J, Gray CM, Rademeyer C, Seoighe C, Ramjee G, Karim SA et al (2004) Incidence of HIV-1 dual infection and its association with increased viral load set point in a cohort of HIV-1 subtype C-infected female sex workers. J Infect Dis 190:1355–1359
23. Hu DJ, Subbarao S, Vanichseni S, Mock PA, Ramos A, Nguyen L et al (2005) Frequency of HIV-1 dual subtype infections, including intersubtype superinfections, among injection drug users in Bangkok, Thailand. AIDS 19:303–308
24. Hemelaar J, Gouws E, Ghys PD, Osmanov S (2006) Global and regional distribution of HIV-1 genetic subtypes and recombinants in 2004. AIDS 20:W13–W23
25. Braitstein P, Brinkhof MW, Dabis F, Schechter M, Boulle A, Miotti P et al (2006) Mortality of HIV-1-infected patients in the first year of antiretroviral therapy: comparison between low-income and high-income countries. Lancet 367:817–824
26. Essex M (2009) HIV variability in Africa. In: Kanki P, Marlink R (eds) A line drawn in the sand: responses to the AIDS treatment crisis in Africa. Harvard Center for Population and Development Studies, Cambridge, MA, pp 245–258
27. Ivers LC, Kendrick D, Doucette K (2005) Efficacy of antiretroviral therapy programs in resource-poor settings: a meta-analysis of the published literature. Clin Infect Dis 41: 217–224

28. Kantor R, Katzenstein D (2003) Polymorphism in HIV-1 non-subtype B protease and reverse transcriptase and its potential impact on drug susceptibility and drug resistance evolution. AIDS Rev 5:25–35

29. Vergne L, Peeters M, Mpoudi-Ngole E, Bourgeois A, Liegeois F, Toure-Kane C et al (2000) Genetic diversity of protease and reverse transcriptase sequences in non-subtype-B human immunodeficiency virus type 1 strains: evidence of many minor drug resistance mutations in treatment-naive patients. J Clin Microbiol 38:3919–3925

30. Chaplin B, Eisen G, Idoko J, Onwujekwe D, Idigbe E, Adewole I et al (2010) Impact of HIV type 1 subtype on drug resistance mutations in nigerian patients failing first-line therapy. AIDS Res Hum Retrovir 15:1413–1420

31. Holguin A, Sune C, Hamy F, Soriano V, Klimkait T (2006) Natural polymorphisms in the protease gene modulate the replicative capacity of non-B HIV-1 variants in the absence of drug pressure. J Clin Virol 36:264–271

32. Van De Vijver DA, Wensing AM, Angarano G, Asjo B, Balotta C, Boeri E et al (2006) The calculated genetic barrier for antiretroviral drug resistance substitutions is largely similar for different HIV-1 subtypes. J Acquir Immune Defic Syndr 41:352–360

33. Taiwo B, Chaplin B, Penugonda S, Meloni S, Akanmu S, Gashau W et al (2010) Suboptimal etravirine activity is common during failure of nevirapine-based combination antiretroviral therapy in a cohort infected with non-B subtype HIV-1. Curr HIV Res 8:194–198

34. Doualla-Bell F, Avalos A, Brenner B, Gaolathe T, Mine M, Gaseitsiwe S et al (2006) High prevalence of the K65R mutation in human immunodeficiency virus type 1 subtype C isolates from infected patients in Botswana treated with didanosine-based regimens. Antimicrob Agents Chemother 50:4182–4185

35. Brenner B, Turner D, Oliveira M, Moisi D, Detorio M, Carobene M et al (2003) A V106M mutation in HIV-1 clade C viruses exposed to efavirenz confers cross-resistance to non-nucleoside reverse transcriptase inhibitors. AIDS 17:F1–F5

36. Eshleman SH, Guay LA, Wang J, Mwatha A, Brown ER, Musoke P et al (2005) Distinct patterns of emergence and fading of K103N and Y181C in women with subtype A vs. D after single-dose nevirapine: HIVNET 012. J Acquir Immune Defic Syndr 40:24–29

37. Arrive E, Newell ML, Ekouevi DK, Chaix ML, Thiebaut R, Masquelier B et al (2007) Prevalence of resistance to nevirapine in mothers and children after single-dose exposure to prevent vertical transmission of HIV-1: a meta-analysis. Int J Epidemiol 36:1009–1021

38. Phillips AN, Dunn D, Sabin C, Pozniak A, Matthias R, Geretti AM et al (2005) Long term probability of detection of HIV-1 drug resistance after starting antiretroviral therapy in routine clinical practice. AIDS 19:487–494

39. Seyler C, Adje-Toure C, Messou E, Dakoury-Dogbo N, Rouet F, Gabillard D et al (2007) Impact of genotypic drug resistance mutations on clinical and immunological outcomes in HIV-infected adults on HAART in West Africa. AIDS 21:1157–1164

40. Bussmann H, Novitsky V, Wester W, Peter T, Masupu K, Gabaitiri L et al (2005) HIV-1 subtype C drug-resistance background among ARV-naive adults in Botswana. Antivir Chem Chemother 16:103–115

41. Gordon M, De Oliveira T, Bishop K, Coovadia HM, Madurai L, Engelbrecht S et al (2003) Molecular characteristics of human immunodeficiency virus type 1 subtype C viruses from KwaZulu-Natal, South Africa: implications for vaccine and antiretroviral control strategies. J Virol 77:2587–2599

42. Koizumi Y, Ndembi N, Miyashita M, Lwembe R, Kageyama S, Mbanya D et al (2006) Emergence of antiretroviral therapy resistance-associated primary mutations among drug-naive HIV-1-infected individuals in rural western Cameroon. J Acquir Immune Defic Syndr 43:15–22

43. Konings FA, Zhong P, Agwara M, Agyingi L, Zekeng L, Achkar JM et al (2004) Protease mutations in HIV-1 non-B strains infecting drug-naive villagers in Cameroon. AIDS Res Hum Retrovir 20:105–109

44. Vidal N, Mulanga C, Bazepeo SE, Mwamba JK, Tshimpaka J, Kashi M et al (2006) HIV type 1 pol gene diversity and antiretroviral drug resistance mutations in the Democratic Republic of Congo (DRC). AIDS Res Hum Retrovir 22:202–206

45. Little SJ, Holte S, Routy JP, Daar ES, Markowitz M, Collier AC et al (2002) Antiretroviral-drug resistance among patients recently infected with HIV. New Engl J Med 347:385–394
46. Wensing AM, Van De Vijver DA, Angarano G, Asjo B, Balotta C, Boeri E et al (2005) Prevalence of drug-resistant HIV-1 variants in untreated individuals in Europe: implications for clinical management. J Infect Dis 192:958–966

Chapter 6
A Practical Way to Improve Access to Essential Medicines Against Major Infectious Diseases

Yiming Shao

Introduction

In the globalized world of the twenty-first century, diseases have spread faster than ever before, aided by high-speed air travel and the trade in goods and services between countries and continents [1]. Collaboration between, especially, developed and developing countries, to ensure the availability of technical and other resources is a crucial factor in building and strengthening public health capacity, networks, and systems that strengthen global public health security. Such collaboration could prevent the rapid spread of disease. It is estimated that 2.1 billion airline passengers traveled in 2006; a disease outbreak or epidemic in any part of the world is only a few hours away from becoming an imminent threat somewhere else [2]. Developing countries, which collectively shelter over three quarters of the world's population, face severe public health crises from both widespread infectious diseases, such as HIV epidemics, rampant TB, malaria, and viral hepatitis as well as staggering chronic diseases, such as cardiovascular disease and malignant tumors. Approximately 15 million people die each year due to infectious diseases—predominately in developing countries [3]. The rapid progress of science and technology in the twentieth century uncovered many new forms of medicine, which greatly improved people's health in developed countries. However, patent protection for medical drugs and patent monopoly, as stipulated by the World Trade Organization's (WTO) Agreement on Trade-Related Aspects of Intellectual Property Rights (TRIPS), guarantee monopolizing profits. Essentially, this guarantee causes the price of patent drugs to skyrocket, which severely hinders the accessibility of drugs that are essential to public health in developing countries.

The author acknowledges the contributions of Hong Zhu, Tao Teng, and Yinqi Wu.

Y. Shao (✉)
State Key Laboratory for Infectious Disease Prevention and Control, National Center for AIDS/STD Control and Prevention, Chinese Center for Disease Control and Prevention, Beijing, China
e-mail: yshao08@gmail.com

Y. Lu et al. (eds.), *HIV/AIDS Treatment in Resource Poor Countries: Public Health Challenges*, DOI 10.1007/978-1-4614-4520-3_6,
© Springer Science+Business Media New York 2013

After TRIPS was signed, member countries of the WTO, especially the developing countries, were faced with increasing public health crises and have been persistently seeking a new balance between patent protection and the public health interest of providing essential medicine to their citizens. It is clear that the old WTO regulation and TRIPS agreement actually prevent developing countries from getting essential medicines and also hinder their capability to handle the frequent attacks of emerging infectious diseases. Further development and policy advancement of the WTO regulations are needed to establish a new balance between the protection of intellectual property of medicines and the interests of public health.

From TRIPS to the Doha Declaration: Building a Consensus Between Drug Patent Protection and Public Health Interest

Recent economic globalization and market growth has drawn attention to the role of intellectual property in international trade. As major exporters of these products, developed countries advocate the protection of intellectual property while developing countries worry that intellectual property rights only support the monopoly led by international companies and raise the price of the drugs and total medical costs, ultimately having a negative impact on public health emergency response capability. In 1995, the TRIPS agreement was implemented in Uruguay Round to join the protection of intellectual property rights and the cross-retaliation system of the General Agreement of Tariffs and Trade (GATT). Developing countries agreed to protect intellectual property in exchange for market access and trade preferences from developed countries. In particular, the U.S. used its economic hegemony, along with the trade preference "Carrot" and the big-stick policy of "Super 301 sanctions of penalty article" to force other countries to accept the TRIPS agreement [4], causing conflict over the protection of intellectual property and the right to obtain essential medicines.

After over 5 years of debate and negotiations with pressure from the governments of mainly in developing countries and nongovernmental organizations, a consensus was reached. The Doha Declaration on the TRIPS Agreement and Public Health (simply referred to as the "Doha Declaration") was adopted in November of [5]. It states that the "TRIPS Agreement does not and should not prevent Members from taking measures to protect public health. Accordingly, while reiterating our commitment to the TRIPS Agreement, we affirm that the Agreement can and should be interpreted and implemented in a manner supportive of WTO members' rights to protect public health and, in particular, to promote access to medicines for all" [6]. Therefore, the Doha Declaration reaffirms the right of WTO member states to grant compulsory licenses in a state of national emergency. Compulsory licensing refers to a government's consent to someone other than the patent owner to produce the patented product or process without the consent of the patent owner. Specifically in the medical field, the term denotes the government allowing a third party to produce patented drugs. However, TRIPS mandates that the drugs produced under a compulsory license must be used only in the domestic market, which creates a major obstacle for the countries with no manufacturing capacity in the pharmaceutical sector to import unregistered generic drugs [6].

In November 2003, the WTO Ministerial Conference announced the 2003 General Council's decision on the TRIPS Agreement and Public Health (a General Council decision) and included an amendment to paragraph (f) of Article 31 of the TRIPS Agreement. The first revision of the series waived the obligations of exporting members: generic drugs produced under compulsory licenses can be exported to other developing countries lacking the manufacturing capacity instead of remaining exclusive to the domestic market within the manufacturing country. This additional stipulation to the law removed obstacles hindering developing countries' ability to make full use of compulsory licenses. The second revision waived the remuneration to patent holders from importing countries because the exporting country already pays it. This General Council decision resolved the previous issues of paragraph 6 of the Doha Declaration. As a result, member states lacking manufacturing capacity found themselves with the means to import cheap generic drugs from countries that produced the drugs under compulsory licenses.

In December 2005, the WTO General Council adopted the Protocol Amending the TRIPS Agreement, which was the first amendment to TRIPS since 1995 [7]. Up to now, many developing and developed countries have approved the Protocol Amending the TRIPS Agreement. Developing countries should make full use of the privileges introduced by this document by granting compulsory licenses in public health related areas or use it as a tool to acquire a voluntary license in the local manufacture of drugs or in negotiation for affordable drug price. These areas should target drugs for prevention and treatment of infectious diseases and tumors, including HIV/AIDS, hepatitis B, as well as malignant tumors, to break the high price barrier of imported patent drugs and make them accessible to the respective country's population. This direction, if taken, will significantly minimize these serious public health issues in China as well as in other developing countries.

The Implementation of Compulsory Licenses in Developing Countries: A Case Study

WTO treaties, including the Doha Declaration, the General Council Decision, and the Protocol Amending the TRIPS Agreement, stipulate that member countries have the right to grant compulsory licenses and provide necessary legal foundations for member countries to implement compulsory licenses. The treaties specify to what extent a compulsory license may be applied and exactly what constitutes a national emergency. Some developing countries, including Thailand, Brazil, South Africa, and a few others, have already made full use of compulsory licenses to deal with the public health crises posed by infectious diseases such as HIV/AIDS. Refer to Table 6.1 for information on the implantation of compulsory licenses in developing countries [10].

Table 6.1 The implementation of compulsory license in developing countries

Country	Type	Type of drugs
Asia		
India	Compulsory license	All drugs prior to January 1st, 2005. Drugs with a patent (about 8,296 patent drugs) submitted between 1995 and 2005, including some second-line antiretroviral drugs
Malaysia	Compulsory license	AIDS drugs
Indonesia	Compulsory license	AIDS drugs
Thailand	Compulsory license	AIDS drugs, anticancer drugs, cardiovascular medicine
Africa		
Zambia	Compulsory license	AIDS drugs
Mozambique	Compulsory license	AIDS drugs
Zimbabwe	Compulsory license	AIDS drugs
South Africa	Extended the importation, manufacture, and voluntary licensing to other African countries of antiretroviral drugs in four generic drug companies in South Africa	AIDS drugs
Cameroon	Granted public procurement agencies the right to purchase antiretroviral generic drugs when the price is lower than that of the patent owners	AIDS drugs
Ghana	Compulsory license	AIDS drugs
Eritrea	Compulsory license	AIDS drugs
Guinea	Compulsory license	AIDS drugs
Latin America		
Peru	Compulsory license	AIDS drugs
Brazil	Compulsory license	AIDS drugs
China		
China	Threaten to use compulsory license	Oseltamivir phosphate
Taiwan	Compulsory license	CD-R and oseltamivir phosphate

Brazil

In 2005, Brazil began negotiations to issue a compulsory license for kaletra (a second-line antiretroviral drug). Eventually the threat of this compulsory license led to an agreement with the patent holder, Abbott, to reduce the price of the drug [8].

The Brazilian government has consistently sought lower prices for antiretroviral (ARV) drugs in order to support the cost of its national AIDS treatment program, which provides free access to ARV drugs for up to 180,000 Brazilians. It is estimated that 75,000 of those receiving ARV treatment in Brazil will be using efavirenz by the end of 2007. Efavirenz (in tablets of 600 mg) was sold in Brazil at $580 per patient per year, which was 136% higher than the price offered by

Thailand [9]. The Brazilian government attempted negotiations for a lower price with Merck beginning in November 2006. They threatened Merck with a compulsory license unless Brazil could sell efavirenz at a rate equal to or less than the rate offered to Thailand.

After 6 months of unsuccessful negotiations, the Brazilian government issued their first compulsory license on May 4, 2007. Brazil reduced the price per day from $1.56 to $0.45 by buying Indian generic products. The government expected to save $30 million in 2007 and a total of $237 million between 2007 and 2012. "From an ethical point of view the price difference is grotesque," said Brazilian President Luiz Inacio Lula da Silva. "And from a political point of view, it represents a lack of respect, as though a sick Brazilian is inferior," he added. "Our decision today involves this one drug, but we can take the same steps with any other that we consider necessary."

Brazilian's nongovernmental organizations (NGOs) are in strong support of this governmental action. The Working Group on Intellectual Property of the Brazilian Network has said that the government will no longer be a "Tiger without Teeth." The issuance of a compulsory license was an historical decision helping to maintain the access to necessary medicines.

James Love of Knowledge Ecology International predicted "Brazil and Thailand's large expansion of their market for generic versions of Efavirenz, will promote reduced prices, eventually reaching less than $0.24 per day" [10]. Love also added, "Brazil should set up a system of collective management of intellectual property rights and extend a compulsory license for all prescription medicines, not only for AIDS but also for other important health problems like diabetes, cancer, or heart disease."

South Africa

The government of South Africa first issued a compulsory license in 1998 after the TRIPS agreement came into effect. HIV infected 15% of all South Africans and the HIV prevalence among its adult population was as high as 20%, among the highest in the world [11]. In response to the severe epidemic, South Africa passed the *South Africa Medicines and Related Substances Act* in December 1997, authorizing the government to issue a compulsory license and parallel importation. In February 1998, a South African pharmaceutical group united 40 companies who, together, filed a lawsuit on the claim that the *South Africa Medicines and Related Substances Act* of 1997 is unconstitutional because it gives the Minister of Public Health the power to ignore the Patent Act. Ultimately, these companies faced an ethical dilemma of protecting patents over saving human lives and finally withdrew the lawsuit and substantially reduced the price of the drugs. In response, the multinational pharmaceutical companies pressured their own governments asking them to amend the TRIPS Agreement. This action resulted in the Doha Declaration on the TRIPS Agreement and the protocol amending TRIPS [12].

On September 19, 2002, the Treatment Action Campaign and South Africa's Competition Commission filed a lawsuit against GlaxoSmithKline and Boehringer Ingelheim. These two companies were accused of charging exorbitant prices for ritonavir, lamivudine, and nevirapine. GlaxoSmithKline and Boehringer Ingelheim were also found guilty of violating the Competition Act of 1998, abusing their high-standing positions in the ARV markets, denying competitors access to an essential facility, and engaging in an exclusionary act. The terms of the final settlement required the two pharmaceutical companies to extend the voluntary license granted to Aspen Pharmacare to the public and private sectors in October of 2001. This action granted up to three more voluntary licenses on the same terms as those given to Aspen Pharmacare, permitted the export of ARVs to sub-Saharan African countries, and charged royalties of no more than 5% of the net sales of the relevant ARV drugs. This settlement marked an historic victory in the struggle of developing countries fighting against multinational pharmaceutical enterprises using the patent to establish a profitable monopoly over the industry [13].

Thailand

Brief History

Towards the end of 2006, The government of Thailand granted compulsory licenses for two ARV drugs (efavirenz–lopinavir and kaletra) as well as plavix for cardiovascular disease at the end of 2006 and early 2007. In September 2007, the National Drugs Protection Office in Thailand announced its intention to grant compulsory licenses for four cancer drugs: glivec and femara from Novartis, tarceva from Roche, and taxotere from Sanofi–Aventis. In January 2008, the compulsory licenses were granted to femara, tarceva, and taxotere. Glivec was exempt because Novartis had promised to provide glivec free of charge to cancer patients inside the Thai National Health Insurance Program [14].

Compulsory Licenses in Thailand

Thailand has a severe HIV/AIDS epidemic. According to (UNAIDS) 2010 Global AIDS Report, there were 530,000 people living with HIV/AIDS and 12,000 new infections in 2009. The prevalence among adults is less than 1.3% [15]. The epidemic has undergone three phases: low epidemic in 1984–1990, rapid increase in 1990–1997, rapid decline from 1997 to the present. The curb of the epidemic is mainly due to the comprehensive measures of public education, prevention, and treatment adopted by Thai government [16, 17]. Despite increased funding from the government, they are still far from meeting the patients' needs and the expensive patent drugs remain a heavy financial toll on the Thai government.

Efavirenz, which is recommended by the World Health Organization (WHO) for HIV/AIDS treatment, has been named one of the best components for first and second line therapy. The price from Merck was $468 per patient per year, which was more than double the price of Indian generics. With Merck's original price, the Thai Ministry of Health (MOH) was only able to cover two-thirds of the population in need. After failed negotiations with Merck [18, 19], the Thai government issued a compulsory license for efavirenz on December 6, 2006, and began the local production with the government pharmaceutical organization (GPO). The price of the drug dropped about 50% from $67 to $38.5 per month [20]. This was the first time Thailand used a strategy permitted under both patent law and the Protocol Amending the TRIPS Agreement.

Lessons Learned

There are two lessons to be learned from the Thai practice of compulsory license. One is the Thai government's planning and coordination to overcome various barriers and challenges, including a remarkably orderly implementation of the "government use" system. The Thai MOH established a government committee directing the government agency's work on compulsory license to ensure that the drugs obtained through the compulsory license are on the national essential list for government use based on Article 51 of Thailand's Patent Act of 1979, which stated that the government can sue the patent owner's rights as their own under certain conditions. The committee broadened the special conditions for public use of compulsory license drugs to include the following:

• To resolve the public health issues
• To be used in emergency situations
• To prevent the infection disease outbreaks
• To save lives

Thai Ministry of Health committee also successfully used a compulsory license as an effective tool to lower the price for other ARV drugs.

From 2004 to 2006, the Thai government was actively negotiating the price of Kaletra with Abbott. In 2006, Abbott initially offered a rate of $2,976 per patient per year [21]. After being pressured by the Thai MOH and NGOs, Abbott lowered the offer to $1,000 and declared no further price reduction. Because kaletra's cost of production was less than $400, the Thai MOH decided to issue a compulsory license. Abbott responded by arguing that the Thai government was ignoring the patent law and threatened to withdraw registration of all new drugs in Thailand. However, the WHO along with many other individual countries and NGOs affirmed that the movement of issuing compulsory licenses was consistent with International Law. In 2007, Thailand and other developing countries succeeded in reducing the price of generic kaletra to $676 per patient per year [22].

The Practice of Compulsory Licenses in Developed Countries

Developed countries such as the USA and Canada have also made full use of compulsory licenses in the field of public health to maintain the national interests and solve public crises according to the Protocol Amending TRIPS. In October 2001, there was a nationwide anthrax scare in USA resulting in rising demands for ciprofloxacin (Cipro). Anecdotally, many health professionals believe that "it is not anthrax, but the price of the drugs for anthrax that caused the panic." The US government was faced with a dilemma during the 2001 anthrax scare. The US government consistently supported intellectual property protection for large pharmaceutical companies. Therefore, issuing a compulsory license for Cipro was a controversial act. In the end, the US government used the threat of a compulsory license to force Bayer to significantly lower its price and thus saved $276 million [23].

From 2005 to 2007, the Italian government issued a compulsory license for three drug types, including an anti-infection antibiotic, a drug for the treatment of migraine headaches, and a prostate drug. The Italian government also authorized the export of these drugs to other EU member states. These actions are countermeasures to prevent monopolies under the provisions of Article 40 in the Protocol Amending the TRIPS agreement (James 2007).

Unlike the decisions of the US and Italian governments to use a compulsory license for their own interests, Canada, the first country to amend its domestic intellectual property laws according to the 2003 General Council's decision on the TRIPS Agreement, used the compulsory license for the purpose of helping people in developing countries to obtain urgently needed medicines. Canada's Access to Medicines Regime (CAMR) was drafted in May 2004 and became effective in May 2005 [24]. CAMR requested the generic drug producer first negotiate voluntary licensing from the patent holder before issuing the compulsory license. After failed negotiation with GlaxoSmithKline and Boehringer Ingelheim, for a voluntary license and with petition from Rwanda to the World Trade Organization, Canada granted the Apotex company a compulsory license for TriAvir in [25] to be exported to Rwanda [26].

The Urgent Demand for Generic Drugs in Developing Countries

Generic Drug Demands for Infectious Diseases

The epidemics of AIDS, tuberculosis, malaria, and other major infectious diseases and the shortage of treatment drugs and preventive vaccines are the most serious public health problems in developing countries. Due to the lack of effective medicines and necessary medical intervention, infectious diseases in developing countries threaten global public health security. WHO officers pointed out that in many developing countries, especially in Africa, the major issue is finding a way to import drugs for infectious diseases as soon as possible.

According to Joint United Nations Programme on HIV/AIDS [15] Global AIDS Report, there were 33 million people infected with HIV in the world, with over 90% in developing countries, including 22.5 million people living in sub-Saharan Africa [15]. WHO, UNICEF, and UNAIDS reported that there were 14 million AIDS patients and HIV infected people needing ARV treatment. However, only 30% of them received the necessary medications [27]. Recently published research demonstrated that early ARV treatment in discordant couples and preexposure drug prophylaxis in MSM (men who have sex with men) can significantly reduce HIV transmission. These findings will greatly increase the demand for ARV drugs in the near future.

According to the WHO data in 2010 [28], there were 8.8 million TB cases, 1.1 million TB deaths in HIV-negative populations, and an additional 0.35 million deaths in HIV-positive populations. In 2010, there were 5.7 million notifications of new and recurrent cases of TB, equivalent to 65% of the estimated number of incident cases. India and China accounted for 40% of the world's reported TB cases, Africa for another 24%, and the 22 countries with the highest TB rates accounted for 82%. Fewer than 5% of new and previously treated TB patients were tested for multidrug-resistant tuberculosis (MDR-TB) in most countries. The reported number of patients enrolled in MDR-TB treatment has increased, reaching 46,000. However, this was equivalent to only 16% of the 290,000 cases of MDR-TB estimated to exist among reported TB patients in 2010.

China is one of the 22 countries characterized as having a severe TB epidemic, ranking the second after India. There are 1.3 million patients diagnosed with a TB infection, comprising up to 14.3% of the global incidence and 80% of which are from rural areas, especially the northwest part of China where the economy is least developed [29]. The MDR-TB epidemic in China is very severe and accounts for 1/4–1/3 of the global incidence and is listed by WHO as one of the countries/regions requiring special attention [30]. All drugs available for MDR or XDR TB (extensively drug-resistant tuberculosis) are brand drugs manufactured by the big pharmaceutical companies in developed countries.

The 2009 WHO World Malaria Report [31] indicated that 3.3 billion people globally are threatened by malaria, exceeding half of the world's population. Each year, there are about 250 million cases of malaria, 85% of which are in Africa with the majority being children. The most severely hit populations are in sub-Saharan Africa with an average of 3,000 children under the age of 5 dying from malaria each day. There is limited access to antimalaria treatment, especially the artemisinin-based combination cocktail medicine, in Africa. In 2007–2008, 11 of the 13 African countries with available data showed that less than 15% of population under the age of 5 with a fever received the combination cocktail medicine. In 2008, the public health facilities in some African countries could only meet half of the demand for antimalaria medicines.

Hepatitis B virus (HBV) has one of the highest morbidity rates and is sometimes referred to as the "second cancer." There are 350 million patients with chronic HBV infection globally, 30–40% of which are chronic HBV patients. China is greatly affected by this epidemic, currently with 120 million chronic HBV infection cases and 3 million chronic HBV patients. It is estimated that the total direct and indirect loss due to chronic Hepatitis B (including Hepatocirrhosis and Hepatocellular Carcinoma) costs 90 billion Chinese RMB each year [32]. Since all antiviral drugs for HBV and HCV are imported brand drugs, most people in developing countries, including China, cannot afford to use the antiviral drugs for their treatment.

A Case Study of the Chinese Pharmaceutical Industry

There is a high demand for medicine in developing countries. These demands are increasing each year, especially in countries such as China and India with rapid development and improving living standards. In China, Mr. Mingde Yu, President of the China Pharmaceutical Enterprises Association disclosed that because of the recent spike in demand for medical drugs and medical reform, the market share for common medicine has increased to over 160 billion RMB [33]. The annual growth of the pharmaceutical industry in China is expected to be at 30%. It is estimated that the total pharmaceutical sales in China will amount to US$46 billion in 2011 with China as the third largest pharmaceutical industry after the USA and Japan [34]. A survey conducted by CSPS Parma in the top-notch hospitals (the AAA level in the Chinese Hospital grade system) in Beijing and Shanghai showed that foreign and imported medicines comprise 97% of sales and that the top 100 drugs used in those hospitals are all imported drugs. The gross output of China's pharmaceutical industry was 866.68 billion RMB in 2008. The total incomes of the medical and pharmaceutical industry were 778.79 billion RMB, with 449 billion RMB from chemical drugs, biological drugs, and traditional Chinese medicines. In contrast, the gross sale of joint venture and foreign enterprises was about 200 billion RMB, comprising 35–45% of China's market [35]. Essentially, half of China's pharmaceutical market was controlled by the foreign companies.

Statistics also showed that the market expansion for the domestic pharmaceutical industry was about 10% while it was 40% for the international pharmaceutical companies, mostly due to the patented drugs. Patented drugs usually are a dozen times more expensive than the generic drugs. Patented drugs only comprise about 5% of all drug usage in China, but make up over 20% of sales of the total drug market. To promote universal medical coverage, generic drugs are invariably a better choice for China and other developing countries.

Generic Drug Production Capacity in Developing Countries

Generic Drug Factories and their Capability in Developing Countries

China and India are among the largest global producers of generic drugs and play a major role in providing essential drugs to their people, including more than one-third of the world's total population. China is the largest producer and exporter of

API (Active Pharmaceutical Ingredients) supplies [36] to many multinational pharmaceutical companies and takes up half of the global API market share for many antiviral drugs. According to incomplete statistics, the USA is China's largest purchaser of API. Most of the common antibiotics API in Europe also come from China and India [37].

The four largest API manufacturers for ARV drugs in China could supply almost all of the current ARV drugs worldwide. Their annual production capacity is 7,690 tons, with 60–70% exported and with India as the largest purchaser, followed by western pharmaceutical companies. In response to the low demand of the Chinese for antiviral drugs, the four companies recently developed limited manufacturing capabilities of four to five off-patent ARV drugs. The annual production capacity of these four companies is 96 billion pills. Due to the small domestic market, the sale capacity was less than 1% of production capacity [38]. China has about 5,000 pharmaceutical companies and about 10% are on a similar scale to the above four companies. Many of them also have dual operations with majority API exported and medical drugs mainly sold in the domestic market. Chinese companies have developed many generic drugs including the popular three-ARV drug combination pill. Due to the patent issues, China's State Food and Drug Administration (SFDA) does not accept generic drug applications for these drugs under patent protection. The small domestic market and the patent obstacles of the international market have severely restricted the ability of the Chinese pharmaceutical companies to satisfy the huge demands for essential medicines both at home and in other developing countries.

The Chinese companies hope that the government can implement compulsory licenses to improve their situation. In their opinion, if the country issues compulsory licenses, the generic ARV drugs they manufacture can be exported, which will expand the country's production capacity and further reduce the cost of the ARV drugs. For instance, the price of lamivudine (3TC) could be reduced to one-tenth of the current price in China and nevirapine to one-tenth of its international price. Trizivir would only cost 1,000 Chinese RMB per year per person, which is two-fifths of the lowest international price. The companies promise to provide free ARV drugs for the national treatment program once they gain access to the international market [38].

The Major Role of the Indian Pharmaceutical Industry in the Global Market

The recent astounding rise of Indian pharmaceutical industry has made it the leading industry in the country. India ranks fourth in the global pharmaceutical market [39]. The swift rise of Indian pharmaceutical industry is greatly due to the production of generic drugs. Reddy, an Indian pharmaceutical company, started by producing API for Ibuprofen and exporting API of Methyldopa to Germany in 1986. Its API production passed SFDA (should be FDA?) certification in 1987–1990. Reddy set up distribution centers in America and France in 1992 and 1993. By 2005, 56 products passed the US Food and Drug Administration (FDA) certification with a sales revenue reaching US$175 million. After 4 years of effort, Reddy's production facility for Ranitidine (a nonpatent drug) passed the FDA certification in 1998, and the gateway for medical drugs to developed countries was opened. Currently, 35 of Reddy's nonpatent drugs have passed the FDA certification. The company also owns many distribution sites in America (with headquarters in New Jersey) and Europe (with headquarters in England). Other Indian companies, such as Ranbaxy and Cipla, have gone through similar development paths [40].

India is arguably the largest generic product production country in the world. It houses more than 20,000 pharmaceutical companies, around 260 of which are large-scale companies. India can produce nearly all popular domestic medicines and around 350 common medicines, which meets 70% of its domestic needs. Indian medicine accounts for 8% of the global medicine sales volume. It is the fifth largest producer of APIs worldwide, with an estimated market value of $0.8 billion and is increasing at the rate of 13.4% per year [39].

Meanwhile, India is the largest exporter of nonpatent drugs; 40% of its products are exported to more than 100 countries [40]. Presently, the export revenue of most Indian pharmaceutical companies accounts for more than half of their total revenue. Indian pharmaceuticals companies now account for 20% of American generic drug market share.

By 2000, the exportation value of Indian generic products had reached $1.6 billion [41]. In 2008, the confederation of the Indian pharmaceutical industry reported that medicine exportation accounted for 4.1% of all Indian exportation, and forecasted that the generic product exportation would reach US$10 billion by 2010 [42]. The International Aid Institution Oxfam reveals that more than two-thirds of Indian generic medicine is exported to other developing countries, and that the successful operation of the UN Children's Fund, Médecins Sans Frontières, and other aid efforts rely on the low cost of Indian generic pharmaceutical products [43].

Lessons Learned from the Indian Pharmaceutical Industry

The success of the Indian generic drugs is greatly attributed to the Indian governmental support, its unique patent laws, and the government policy. Indian premier Rajiv Gandhi once said, "Medical inventions are not patented, and we cannot make profits between life and death." The patent law issued in 1970 declared that food, medicine, agricultural chemicals cannot be patented; only the method of making these products can be patented. Therefore, one can make the same exact product or drug by a different methodology according to the Indian Patent Law. This regulation was vital to the rise of the Indian domestic pharmaceutical industry. For many years, the Indian government has withstood pressure from western countries and maintained efficient laws for generic production on the grounds of promoting health and equity. After its entrance into the WTO in 1995, India was pressured by western countries to enter the TRIPS agreement but was granted a period of 10 years to adapt their patent laws to the international standards. India issued the 2004 Patent (amendment) Bill on December 26, 2004. This law mandates that India must begin accepting medicine, agricultural chemicals, and food patent applications from January 1, 2005. However, the Indian government stated that they would only recognize applications submitted from January 1, 1995 onwards and also declared that certain drugs, methods, or applications cannot be patented. At the same time, the Indian Patent Office maintains a unique flexibility in its approval process for generic drugs [44]. For example, if the US FDA has approved a drug, a generic version can be approved for use without first going through a clinical trial in India.

The Indian pharmaceutical industry is at a high level of internationalization. Facing strong foreign competitors, Indian pharmaceutical companies' success is mainly due to their strong entrepreneurship, talented researchers and business development people, and the high quality and low price of their products. India has strategically entered foreign markets by buying up the US and European local pharmaceutical companies. Many Indians are trained in the west and thus fully understand the regulation and the western culture. Their ability to communicate in English also simplifies their international work.

Generic Drug Use in Developed Countries

It is reported in the Journal of the American Medical Association that the U.S. President's Emergency Plan for AIDS Relief (PEPFAR) saved an estimated $323,343,256 from 2005 to 2008 through the use of generic ARV drugs [45]. This significant cost savings contributed to PEPFAR's ability to dramatically improve access to antiretroviral therapy in sub-Saharan Africa and other regions. In 2008, there were eight PEPFAR programs that procured at least 90% of ARV packs in generic form. Additionally, deliveries in Ethiopia, Haiti, Namibia, Rwanda, Tanzania, and Zimbabwe were more than 99% generic. The officer in PEPFAR strongly supported the use of generic drugs because saving money ultimately means saving more lives [45]. One of the biggest hurdles in the rapid scale-up of ARV therapy in developing countries is the high cost of the ARV drugs. However, developed countries in the west and large international pharmaceutical companies are strongly against the compulsory licenses. They often justify their standpoint that they believe it is against patent law to produce generic drugs and that such ability will have a negative impact on the research and development of new drugs. The use of patented drugs is acceptable in developing countries. However, given the current epidemics and public health crises in developing countries, patented drugs are simply inadequate. Generic medications provide an affordable means to provide treatment to more people suffering from HIV/AIDS. In order to solve the demand of patent drugs in developing countries, and to save more lives around the world, the best long-term solution can be provided by compulsory licensing.

Conclusion

Patent protection for medical drugs is a double-edged sword, encouraging discovery of new drugs but at the same time limiting accessibility to patented drugs. The significant polarization of the rich and the poor can be translated to accessibility and inaccessibility of medical drugs, which equates with developed countries and developing countries. Differing from other commodities, drugs are essential for saving lives. The international community has reached a consensus about the conflict between the monopolies protected by patents and public health and has chosen to protect public health and expand the accessibility of drugs. This decision is apparent in the TRIPS agreement adopted by WTO General Council in 2005. Developing countries should use the rights endowed by Protocol Amending the TRIPS agreement and issue compulsory licenses for drugs against major diseases to safeguard the health of their people and public health interests of their nations.

Some developed countries and large pharmaceutical companies had opposed the implementation of a compulsory license practice by developing countries, arguing it might hinder drug discovery research. The truth behind this claim, however, is that governments have the resources to buy the brand drugs. The large pharmaceutical companies lobbying to protect their monopolies also exert a strong influence. However, when there is a public health threat, developed countries will issue compulsory licenses without hesitation to solve the crisis. A good example is the US government forcing Bayer to reduce the price of Cipro using the compulsory licensing as a last resort after the September 11 attack in 2001. A WHO official pointed out that the global economy increases at an annual rate of 1%, much lower than the increase of average drug prices. According to the 2007 OECD report, drugs that took up 6–7% of the health budget of developed countries 10 years ago doubled or tripled their percentage in the health budget today [46]. At the present trend, developed countries may have difficulties affording the high drug prices in the next 10–20 years and may choose compulsory licensing as a tool to solve their health care.

As for developing countries, drug cost takes up a much larger percentage (20–50%) of their limited health expenditure. If strong measures are not taken, the government will be unable to provide enough drugs to its citizens, especially to the vulnerable groups. A tragic example of this occurred in the first 10 years of ARV treatment for HIV/AIDS. While the treatment was widely available in developed countries, AIDS patients in developing countries, which make up more than 90% of the AIDS patients worldwide, were still dying in large numbers. Some developing countries such as Thailand, Brazil, Malaysia, and South Africa took a bold move to provide generic drugs to their AIDS patients through the compulsory licensing. Such acts not only saved many lives, but also eased the burden of high drug costs and prevented the collapse of their national economies. Canada, a developed country and member of the G7, has initiated a compulsory license to provide ARV drugs to the HIV/AIDS patients in Africa.

Countries with large emerging economies, such as India, China, Brazil, and South Africa, are not only faced with the public health challenges of financing essential drugs and vaccines for their huge population but also the responsibility to help other developing countries, especially the least developed countries in Africa, to solve their public health crises. China is the world's largest producer of APIs, including more than half the global APIs used for ARV drugs and antibiotics. India is the world's largest producer for generic drugs. Therefore, it is advantageous for all developing countries to work together for the research, production, and distribution of generic drugs.

Through the PEPFAR and other global health programs, the USA is the largest founder and the major player in the global AIDS, TB, and malaria treatment programs covering African and other developing countries. Most of the ARV drugs used in these US founded programs are actually generic drugs manufactured in developing countries, mostly in India. Additionally, the big pharmaceutical companies in the developed countries developed all of the ARV drugs and most of the anti-TB and malaria drugs. Some of the drugs were developed by developing countries, such as artemisinin, which was invented by the Chinese scientists. Without the close collaborations in the last decade between the south and the north and the private and public, the lives of several millions of HIV/AIDS patients, TB patients, and malaria patients would not have been saved. Therefore, developed countries and big pharmaceutical companies must ally with the developing countries in the war against AIDS, TB, malaria, and other infectious diseases. Due to the lack of such collaboration, the initial sparks of HIV infections in central Africa become a global AIDS pandemic killing 30 million lives in both the developing and developed world. Such tragedy can only be prevented through further strengthening collaboration between the private and public sectors in both developed and developing countries.

References

1. Alirol E et al (2011) Urbanisation and infectious diseases in a globalised world. Lancet Infect Dis 11(2):131–141
2. Stacey K et al (2006) The impact of globalization on infectious disease emergence and control: Exploring the consequences and opportunities, Workshop summary—forum on microbial threats. The National Academies Press, Washington, DC
3. World Trade Organization (2008) WHO global burden of disease: 2004 update. http://www.who.int/healthinfo/global_burden_disease/2004_report_update/en/index.html
4. Ryan MP (1998) The function-specific and linkage-bargain diplomacy of international intellectual property Lawmaking. 19 U. Pa. J. Int'l Econ. L. 535
5. World Trade Organization (2001) The Doha Declaration explained. http://www.wto.org/english/tratop_e/dda_e/dohaexplained_e.htm. Accessed Nov 2001
6. World Trade Organization (2001) TRIPS and public health. http://www.wto.org/english/tratop_e/trips_e/paper_develop_w296_e.htm
7. World Trade Organization (2005) Amendment of the TRIPS agreement. http://www.wto.org/english/tratop_e/trips_e/wtl641_e.htm
8. Alcorn K (2007) Brazil issues compulsory license on efavirenz. Aidsmap News. http://www.aidsmap.com/Brazil-issues-compulsory-license-on-efavirenz/page/1427206/

9. SUNS (2007) Brazil moves on compulsory license after failed talks with drug company. Third world network (TWN). http://www.twnside.org.sg/title2/intellectual_property/info.service/twn.ipr.info.050701.htm. Accessed 1 May 2007
10. Love JP (2007) Recent examples of the use of compulsory license on patents. Knowledge Ecology International. http://accessvector.org/oldkei/content/view/41/
11. Saslow EL (1999) Compulsory licensing and the AIDS epidemic in South Africa. AIDS Patient Care STDs 13(10):577–584
12. Zhang XY (2004) Analysis the system of compulsory license. Master degree thesis, Peking University
13. CPTech (2011) Examples of health-related compulsory licenses http://www.cptech.org/ip/health/cl/recent-examples.html
14. He YX (2008) Thai government committee to review legality of issued compulsory licenses. http://www.sipo.gov.cn/dtxx/gw/2008/200804/t20080401_353860.html. Accessed 12 Mar 2008
15. UNAIDS (2010) Global report: UNAIDS report on the global AIDS epidemic 2010. http://www.unaids.org/globareport/global_report.htm
16. Wattana SJ et al (2002) Perinatal AIDS mortality and orphanhood in the aftermath of the successful control of the HIV epidemics: the case of Thailand, 2002
17. Wiput P (2004) Thailand's response to HIV/AIDS: progress and challenges
18. Cawthorne P et al (2007) WHO must defend patients' interests, not industry. Lancet 369(9566):974–975
19. Gerhardsen TIS (2006) Thailand compulsory license on aids drug prompts policy debate. http://www.ip-watch.org/weblog/index.php?p=499&res=1024_ff&print=0. Accessed 23 Dec 2006
20. Ling CY (2006) Thailand uses compulsory license for cheaper AIDS drug
21. Steinbrook R (2007) Thailand and the compulsory licensing of efavirenz. New Engl J Med 356:544–546
22. Nathan F et al (2007) Sustaining access to antiretroviral therapy in the less-developed world: lessons from Brazil and Thailand. AIDS 21(suppl 4):S21–S29
23. Sun H (2005) Analysis of the compulsory license of patents. Study Times. http://www.netlawcn.net/second/content.asp?no=1358. Accessed 19 Jun 2005
24. Holger PH (2007) Canadian-made drugs for Rwanda: the first application of the WTO waiver on patents and medicines. ASIL Insight 10:2007
25. World Trade Organization (2007) Trips and public health—patents and health: WTO receives first notification under 'Paragraph 6' system. http://www.wto.org/english/news_e/news07_e/public_health_july07_e.htm
26. Kaiser Daily HIV/AIDS Report (2008) Canadian drug company awarded Rwandan contract to provide combination antiretroviral. http://shippa.info/2011/06/canadian-drug-company-awarded-rwandan-contract-to-provide-combination-antiretroviral/
27. World Trade Organization (2008) Towards universal access: scaling up priority HIV/AIDS interventions in the health sector. http://www.who.int/hiv/pub/2008progressreport/en/
28. World Trade Organization (2011) Global tuberculosis control 2011. http://www.who.int/tb/publications/global_report/2011/gtbr11_full.pdf
29. Ministry of Health (2011) Introduction of the national TB epidemic status by Ministry of Health. http://www.moh.gov.cn/publicfiles/business/htmlfiles/mohjbyfkzj/s3590/201103/51027.htm
30. UN News Center (2008) Drug-resistant tuberculosis on the rise, UN health agency says. http://www.un.org/chinese/News/fullstorynews.asp?newsID=9370. Accessed 26 Feb 2008
31. World Trade Organization (2009) World malaria report 2009. http://www.who.int/malaria/world_malaria_report_2009/en/
32. Zhuang H (2005) Chronic hepatitis B prevention and treatment guidelines. Press conference speeches in China. China Foundation for Hepatitis Prevention and Control. http://www.cfhpc.org/detail.asp?ID=81&page=1
33. Zeng LM (2009) Chinese pharmaceutical retail market is growing, and to be 66 billion yuan in the first half year. http://www.chinanews.com/jk/news/2009/11-08/1952968.shtml. Accessed 8 Dec 2009

34. Tan J et al (2009) Chairman of the Pharmaceutical Society of China: China is expected to be the third largest pharmaceutical market in the world. http://news.xinhuanet.com/politics/2009-11/22/content_12521089.htm. Accessed 22 Nov 2009

35. SFDA Southern Medicine Economic Institute (2009) 2009 blue book of development of pharmaceutical market in China. 26 Oct 2009

36. YangCheng Evening Paper (2010) China has become the world's largest raw material medicine producer and exporter. http://news.qq.com/a/20100527/001328.htm

37. LuoXin Company (2011) Several different international export market situation of API in China. http://www.luoxin.cn/newsinfo.asp?id=3446&pid=147

38. Pharmaceutical companies (2010) Pharmaceutical companies' report, 2010

39. Liu N et al (2007) The competitive potential of the Indian pharmaceutical industry. Econ Trade Update 5(70):79–80

40. Li FL et al (2006) The situation and suggestion of Indian pharmaceutical industry. Qilu Pharm Aff 25(8):460–463

41. India Embassy Information Service (2005) Analysis the rising of pharmaceutical industry in India. http://wenku.baidu.com/view/edd1553710661ed9ac51f304.html. Accessed 23 June 2005

42. Mao X (2008) Attention to public health and medical services in India. http://theory.people.com.cn/GB/136457/8243436.html. Accessed 28 Oct 2008

43. Wang LP et al (2007) Who does the patent law protect in India. China Health Industry, 11:84–89

44. Cui LH et al (2007) Strategy response to dilemma in Chinese pharmaceutical industry: based on the balance between generic drugs and patent drugs. Electron Intellect Prop 2007(5):32–35

45. PEPFA (2010) Use of generic antiretroviral drugs and cost savings in U.S. HIV treatment programs. http://www.pepfar.gov/press/releases/2010/144808.htm. Accessed 18 July 2010

46. Germán Velásquez (2009) The global strategies of public health, innovation and intellectual property, speaking report in the training of "The Strategies and Management of Intellectual Property in Public Health, Innovation". Dec 2009

Chapter 7
When Will Most AIDS Patients in the World Have Access to Effective Antiretroviral Therapy?

Yichen Lu

Introduction

In 2002, the Harvard School of Public Health (HSPH) received a grant from the Office of AIDS Research in the US National Institutes of Health (NIH) to pursue the specific goal of helping China to train medical doctors and public health workers in AIDS medical treatment. The following year, HSPH conducted its first AIDS medical training course in Shanghai, China, in collaboration with the National AIDS Center at the Chinese Center for Disease Control and Prevention (CDC) and Fudan University's School of Public Health.

Since then, HSPH has conducted six such training courses and workshops on the same topics in different Chinese cities. The participants in these events usually included a group of renowned Harvard AIDS clinicians who have had many years of working experience not only in the USA but also in developing countries in southern Africa and Southeast Asia. The majority of the trainees were usually doctors from the Chinese countryside, who had worked in small AIDS clinics in rural areas of China. In 2004, HSPH also hosted a group of Chinese AIDS workers on its Boston campus to help them produce a basic medical training manual that they later used to train thousands of village doctors and AIDS workers in Henan province and elsewhere in China. In 2008, the fifth Harvard AIDS Medical Training Course in China included a specific workshop called "AIDS Medical Training in Resource-Poor Countries and Regions: Public Health Challenges." Several speakers from that workshop were subsequently invited to become the contributors to this book. One of the questions repeatedly discussed in these workshops was the title of this chapter: When will most AIDS patients in the world have access to effective antiretroviral (ARV) therapy?

Y. Lu (✉)
Department of Immunology and Infectious Diseases, Harvard School of Public Health, Boston, MA, USA
e-mail: yichenlu@hsph.harvard.edu

Y. Lu et al. (eds.), *HIV/AIDS Treatment in Resource Poor Countries: Public Health Challenges*, DOI 10.1007/978-1-4614-4520-3_7,
© Springer Science+Business Media New York 2013

This is a complicated question without a simple answer. It is also one of the most important questions for public health workers worldwide as AIDS has become—and shall long continue to be—an unavoidable part of our societies. The question eludes a simple answer because most AIDS patients in the world currently do not have the financial capability to pay for the ARV drugs needed for their lifelong treatments. They also live in resource-poor countries or regions that lack the basic health care infrastructures that are essential to support effective ARV therapy. Moreover, as advances in research and treatment change our understandings of "effective ARV therapy," the gap between effective ARV therapies and the capabilities of resource-poor countries to attain them will continue to widen. The definition of an effective ARV therapy in 1999 differed from that of 2009, which will in turn differ from the "effective ARV therapy" of 2019. The lack of basic health care infrastructures in resource-poor countries thus threatens to continually prevent the majority of the world's AIDS patients from receiving the standard of effective care in ARV therapy.

This chapter summarizes various background information and analyses, using material drawn mostly from past HSPH's AIDS Initiatives (HAI) training courses and workshops in China, before offering an answer to its title question.

ARV Drugs

The advent of the effective ARV therapy [1] in 1997 changed AIDS from a fatal infectious disease without a cure to a medically manageable chronic disease. In 2002, within a span of 5 years from the date ARV therapy became widely available in the developed world, the death rate caused by AIDS had declined by about 84% [2]. Unfortunately, this reduced death rate did not extend to AIDS patients who lived outside of developed countries. In fact, more than 90% of AIDS patients worldwide who needed—and continue to need—ARV therapy live in resource-poor countries. They could not and cannot afford ARV drugs, which require lifelong supplies once treatment starts.

Since 1997, an effective ARV therapy has meant very different things to AIDS patients in different countries or regions with different socioeconomic environments. The differences include disparate availabilities of the numbers of the ARV drugs, unequal access to better ARV drug regimens with improved formulations to reduce the drug's side effects and increase the treatment adhesion, and differential access to new clinical diagnosis methods that enable accurate detection of drug-resistant mutants. As discussed in the following sections, an effective ARV therapy requires not only the best ARV drugs suitable for an individual AIDS patient, but also necessary health care infrastructures—including periodical clinical monitoring and medical counseling services. Resource-poor countries and regions have neither the necessary infrastructure nor the ability to pay for the costs of daily ARV drugs. Consequently, those providing ARV drugs to AIDS patients in the developing world must rely on outside financial support from either international funding agencies or

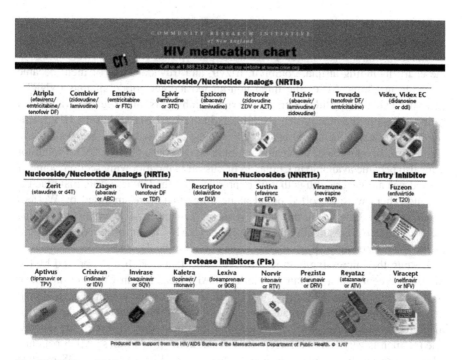

Fig. 7.1 HIV medication chart

national governments. How do such efforts fare? The annual HAI AIDS medical training courses and workshop in China provide a window through which to observe what happened in some of the resource-poor regions in China.

For example, at the beginning series of the training courses, many of our trainees were interested in learning the "common standard" of ARV therapy in the USA Figure 7.1 was one of the slides used in the 2008 Harvard China workshop to address such interests; it shows an HIV medication chart produced by the Community Research Initiative of New England and supported by the Massachusetts Department of Public Health. The chart shows pictures of the different ARV drugs available to the local AIDS patients. At the beginning of the Chinese national ARV therapy program, Chinese AIDS patients had access to only a few of the ARV drugs in the chart; they relied on the free-drug supplies provided by the national government. These drugs included AZT, DDi, D4T, and NVP, all of which were produced by the indigenous Chinese drug manufacturers and approved by the Chinese Food and Drug Administration (SFDA). Although the Chinese national government made these drugs available free of charge to AIDS patients living in underdeveloped provinces and regions in China, the difference between the availability of these drugs in China and their availability in the USA was significant.

The situation in China has changed rapidly in the past several years. By the end of 2010, 21 ARV drugs have received approval from SFDA and have become available to AIDS patients in China. All of the single NRTIs (nucleoside/nucleotide reverse transcriptase inhibitors) in the Massachusetts HIV medication chart in 2007 became available in China 2 years later. There were four types of combined NRTIs drugs in the chart, including atripla, combivir, trizvir, and truvada; three of them became available in China. All of the three non-nucleoside/nucleotide analogs (NNRTI, non-nucleoside/nucleotide reverse transcriptase inhibitors) also became available in China. Seven of the nine protease inhibitors in the 2007 Massachusetts HIV medication chart, which included eight single and one combined drugs, are available in China now. In addition to the fusion inhibitor in the chart, the new CCR5 inhibitor drug also became available in China. As discussed in the following section, some of these drugs are generic drugs that were produced by the Chinese drug manufacturers and others were imported brand name drugs that were imported by Western manufacturers. Judging by this table, it seems that most AIDS patients in China today can receive presumably the same effective ARV treatment as Americans did in 2007. Unfortunately, in reality this turns out not to be the case.

Despite the impressive number of ARV drugs that have been approved by the SFDA in recent years, the supermajority of AIDS patients in China do not have access to most of the ARV drugs that are imported into the country by the brand name drug manufacturers. Because most AIDS patients in China rely on the government to provide the free ARV drugs for their treatment, their choice of the second-line regimen is very limited. Except for a small number of Chinese AIDS patients, who have the financial means to pay for the imported drugs, most AIDS patients still do not have the same access to the ARV drugs listed in the 2007 Massachusetts AIDS medication chart.

There are now more than a dozen of Chinese pharmaceutical companies that have made significant investments to become ARV drug producers and providers. More companies are expected to join. Since the domestic market size of the ARV drugs in China is apparently limited in the near future, what is the financial driving force behind such rapid improvements in the ARV drug availability in China? The answer: the future global market. Although Chinese drug manufacturers currently have very insignificant shares of the global ARV drug market, they supply globally the majority of the active pharmaceutical ingredients (API) for ARV drugs. Over the past several years, this majority has grown annually. The profit margins for these Chinese drug manufacturers to produce API for ARV drugs are actually very low in comparison with producing the drugs directly; however, this picture can change in the coming years if the Chinese national government decides to take similar actions as the governments of India, Thailand, South Africa, and Brazil did in the past decade (more details in Dr. Yiming Shao's chapter of this book).

The most significant obstacle for Chinese pharmaceutical companies to enter the global ARV drug market is the patent protections for the brand name drugs. Any drug manufacturer who wants to produce and sell its products globally must receive the Chinese FDA's approval with regard to its compliances with Good Manufacturing Practices (GMP) regulations. As the national regulatory authority, SFDA is mindful of the fact that the patent protection issues of ARV drug are constantly under the global spotlights with magnifying glasses. For example, despite the fact that many

Chinese drug producers were capable of producing lamivudine in large quantities and with good quality, the SFDA only granted approval in 2008 to one of the major Chinese ARV drug producers, the Shanghai Disaino, after the patent protection for lamivudine in China expired. Soon after that, four more Chinese pharmaceutical companies received SFDA approval, and the export of lamivudine in 2009 increased nearly fivefold within a year [3]. Many of us in the Harvard workshops hoped that in the coming decade when more and more ARV drug patents expire, which include the majority in the 2007 Massachusetts HIV/AIDS medication chart, Chinese pharmaceutical companies will transform from being major API suppliers to ARV drug manufacturers worldwide to being major ARV drug manufacturers themselves. When that happens, it is perhaps possible that one day China can offer affordable, safe, and effective ARV drugs to the world as it does with other made-in-China products.

In many discussions during the HAI workshops in China, participants compared the availability of ARV drugs to that of antibiotics. The advent of successful ARV therapy in 1997 was like the advent of commercial antibiotics in the 1940s: both turned lethal infections into treatable diseases. Like antibiotics, ARV drugs save lives, but only when they are available to patients. We now know that it actually took more than a couple of decades for antibiotics to become widely available throughout the world, especially in developing countries like China. Will it take that long for ARV drugs?

Unlike the antibiotics treatment, the ARV treatment is a lifelong treatment. When an AIDS patient no longer has access to effective ARV drugs — whether due to drug-resistant viruses, or personal financial hardship, or governments' failures to continuously provide the drugs — the disease becomes lethal again. This unique feature of ARV as an anti-infection treatment has become a huge challenge to AIDS patients, to their families, and to the societies in which they live. It is also clear that such a challenge will face future generations as well. HIV/AIDS has become a part of our lives, and each generation of public health workers must do its part to answer the challenges of its time. The challenge we face today seems obvious: making effective ARV drugs available to more AIDS patients.

Necessary Elements for a Government to Provide Effective ARV

When HAI's first China AIDS medical training course was held in Shanghai in 2003, the biggest challenge for most of our trainees was not to learn how to treat AIDS patients with ARV therapy medically, but it was how to overcome the lack of all the necessary health care infrastructure and medical personnel required for effective ARV therapy. In fact, almost all of these necessary health care infrastructures did not exist in 2003 in the resource-poor regions in China, where most of our trainees came from. For example, in most of the villages in Henan province, where the national free-ARV therapies were supposed to start in 2002, there was no trained local clinician or village doctor available at all. The villages also lacked even a place to store the ARV drug supplies, let alone the necessary patient registration and adhesion counsels for ARV therapy.

Prior to the first HAI medical training course in China in 2003, Dr. Max Essex and his colleagues had faced similar challenges in Thailand [4] and Botswana [5] and had successfully collaborated with each country's national public health officials and local public health workers and clinicians. The message we were trying to convey to our Chinese colleagues and trainees in the training courses and workshops was clear: all of these seemingly impossible requirements for effective ARV treatments in resource-poor regions can be met as long as the national and local governments *decide* to provide effective ARV therapy to their AIDS patients.

In the subsequent training courses and workshops in China, we invited a number of key national, provincial, and countryside public health officials who were directly involved with efforts to provide ARV therapy to AIDS patients in poor areas. The following offers a snapshot of what we have witnessed over the past several years in China, based mainly on presentations on building health care infrastructures by Liu Xuezhou (the Deputy director of the Henan provincial department of health), on the effort to identify and treat more AIDS patients in the province by Dr. Cui Zhaolin of the Henan provincial CDC, and on the medical training projects for village doctors by the chief physician of the Henan provincial infectious disease hospital (the 6th people's hospital in Zhengzhou), Dr. Zhao Qingxia.

Building the Necessary Health Care Infrastructures

In 2004, when the AIDS epidemic in Henan province reached a crisis level, the provincial government decided to build the necessary public health infrastructures in order to provide effective ARV treatment to the local AIDS patients, most of whom were farmers who became infected with the virus after selling their plasma for money through illicit medical practices in the previous decade [6]. Since all of these "AIDS villages" (as they were called by the locals because of the high death toll caused by AIDS) were among the poorest villages in the region, the provincial government started the project by assembling the field working groups. These working groups included the deputies or decision-making members of the local banks, major hospitals, and all key branches of the local governments—such as the departments of finance, transportation, public security, education, industrial development—as well as the health department and provincial CDC.

The initial stages of this public health project began with the building of paved roads to the villages so that they could have access to the outside world. As the provincial department of health identified 38 villages in Henan province as villages that urgently needed help to control the AIDS epidemics, 38 field working teams were dispatched who would live and work in each individual village until the initial public health projects were completed. These projects usually sought to establish four elements of a basic public health infrastructure: a paved road, a deep water well, a nursing home for older villagers whose children died of AIDS, and a "care center" for the "AIDS orphans" whose parents died of AIDS.

In order to facilitate the implementation of the national free-ARV treatment, the local governments also had to build many simple "clinics" for these AIDS villages. Such clinics were usually farmhouses, the rooms of which were converted to serve as a doctor's office, a patient's waiting room, and an ARV drug storage rooms for the villages and adjacent farming communities. Since most villages in the region never had any kind of clinic before, and since no medical personnel (such as nurses or trained clinicians) lived in those villages, the new AIDS clinics and the doctors from the provincial capital, nearby cities, or town centers quickly became an attraction to local farmers. As it was necessary for the clinics to provide other minimum medications to treat immune deficiency symptoms caused by AIDS, all AIDS patients enrolled in the free ARV treatment program were issued with a medical ID card to record their treatment histories. Being an AIDS patient in those poor villages suddenly meant having access to some basic health care services that were not available to non-AIDS patients in the same region. As discussed in the next section, this kind of minimum medical service played a significant role in implementing the ARV therapy in the resource-poor regions by attracting otherwise unknown AIDS patients to seek diagnosis and treatment.

Building the paved public roads to the AIDS villages also turned out to be an important factor in the disease control and prevention programs. Among many visible socioeconomic benefits, having access to the outside world by means of any kind of automobile meant that HIV-infected pregnant women could receive periodic counseling and did not have to deliver their babies in homes, thus making it possible to prevent the transmission of HIV from mother to infant.

Public Education Projects

At the first HAI China AIDS medical training course in 2003, one of the biggest concerns on everybody's mind seemed to be the challenges of identifying as many farmers and farmers' family members who were infected with the virus and who needed to be treated with ARV therapies, as possible. From the end of 1990s till the early part of 2000s, the AIDS epidemic in Henan was widely publicized by the news media, especially by international news media. The uniqueness and the special circumstances under which the epidemic spread in the region has been analyzed in depth elsewhere, including in the two previous books published by the editors of this book [4, 7]. The following discussion provides a glance at some of the events that happened in Henan after 2005.

When the AIDS epidemic was first reported to be spreading in the general population in Henan beyond the typically high-risk populations like CSW (commercial sex workers), MSM (men having sex with men), and IDU (intravenous drug users), the biggest worry was how many people had been infected and how to find and treat them medically. Although most of these people were infected by contaminated needles, syringes, and other medical devices used during the illegitimate plasma collection process, they suffered from the same stigmas suffered by people infected with the virus elsewhere in the world. In the face of social stigmas surrounding

HIV/AIDS, most of the local farming community members were afraid of being tested for infection and were very reluctant to accept the free ARV therapy even if they might be very sick due to AIDS. From a public health perspective, the situation was truly worrisome: according to the volumes of the plasma collected in Henan during the 10-year period from 1990 to 2000 and the record of names of the people who sold blood in those contaminated plasma collection centers, the estimated AIDS patients in the province could number in the millions [8].

As the AIDS treatment and prevention program had become a high priority for the provincial government, knowing exactly how many people in the province had been infected and were in need of help would be critical for future government planning in resource allocation and budget forecasting. Finally, in 2005, the provincial government launched an ambitious program focused on identifying and testing everyone who sold blood to the illegitimate commercial plasma trader during the 1990s. At this point, hundreds of village AIDS clinics in the province had started to provide free ARV therapy with trained village doctors or nurses. Dr. Cui Zhaolin of the Henan Provincial CDC presented the results of this project in December 2005, in the 3rd HAI's China AIDS medical training courses, revealing a number of unique features that were unheard of for many of us in attendance. For example, because the cash payment for selling plasma was very attractive to poor farmers who otherwise had little or no commercial activities to make money, the farmers often used other people's names or identities in order to sell their plasma more frequently than they were supposed to (i.e. more than once per week). Consequently, the real number of people who sold plasma during that period was significantly lower than the number of names that appeared on the record books. The provincial government's program also found that in many villages, the commercial activity of selling plasma was so desirable and lucrative that only family members or close friends of some farmers were allowed to participate. Because such practices effectively restricted the actual number of plasma sellers, they in fact lowered the risk of infection resulting from cross-contamination by someone who was infected elsewhere due to high-risk behaviors such as CSW, MSM, or IDU. These findings helped explain why some villages had an HIV infection rate of zero, whereas others had infection rates as high as 50% among past plasma sellers. Many of us believed that public education about HIV/AIDS played an important role in encouraging people to reveal or admit what had actually happened beyond the record keeping.

Medical Training

In providing free ARV therapy to the hundreds of thousands of AIDS patients in regions lacking basic health care infrastructure and trained physicians, the biggest challenge was figuring out how to deliver the free ARV drugs to patients in their homes and how to supervise them to take the medicine properly day by day. Since 2003, thousands of village doctors, most of whom have only had a high school education or the equivalent thereof, went through the basic medical training by the local governments with financial and technical aid from the national and provincial governments. International agencies and organizations such as HAI also helped. For example, a group of Chinese AIDS experts, including representatives from the Chinese national AIDS center, the provincial CDC, the provincial infectious disease hospital, and the AIDS clinic in Wenlou county, visited Harvard with the specific task of producing a basic AIDS medical training manual in Chinese. After their arrival at Boston, they began to translate and modify the field training manuals that had been used success-fully in HAI's previous projects in Thailand and Botswana [9]. They visited differ-ent AIDS clinics in Boston, including those at the Harvard Children's Hospital (Dr. Sandra Burchett), Deaconess Hospital (Dr. Roger Shapiro), and Massachusetts General Hospital (Dr. Marcus Altfeld). As these American doctors had all served as the lecturers in HAI's first AIDS Medical training course in Shanghai and had vis-ited China the previous year, they were able to work closely with the visiting Chinese doctors, and provided much needed first-hand experience and lessons to the prepa-ration of the Chinese AIDS training manual. The Chinese doctors also visited the Fenway Health Care Center (Dr. Ken Meyers) and spent a day in the Boston Back Bay community AIDS care center in Boston.

The first China AIDS medical training course used the "KITSO" [9] manual, which had been used widely in Botswana to train the AIDS medical workers in Africa, as part of its training material. The Chinese visiting doctors collaborated with HAI members such as Dr. Richard Marlink, who was mainly responsible for producing the KITSO manual and managing the medical training in southern Africa. In order to make the manual more applicable to the Henan province, the Chinese visiting doctors had a number of special working sections with several AIDS experts at Harvard Medical School and HSPH to get their help and advice. These faculty experts included Dr. M. Essex (Harvard–Botswana partnership), Dr. Phyllis Kanki (Harvard Nigeria Program), Dr. Jean-Louis Sankale (Harvard Senegal program), and Dr. Marc Lallemant (Harvard Thailand Program). The production and subse-quent revision of the Harvard AIDS Medical Training Manual in Chinese benefited significantly from the active participation of these Harvard researchers, most of whom also served as lecturers at multiple annual HAI medical training courses and workshops in China. Several senior members of the Chinese National ARV Treatment Advisory Group also lectured at HAI's AIDS medical training courses in China, including Dr. She Jie (then the director of the National AIDS Center in Beijing), Dr. Yiming Shao (the chief expert scientist in China CDC), Dr. Zhang Fujie (the director of the national ARV treatment program), as well as Dr. Guixien of Wuhan, Dr. Sun Yongtao of Xi'an, and Dr. Zhao Qingxia of Zhengzhou, who served as members of the HAI China AIDS Medical training program's organizing committee. Many believed that it was the active participation of these famous international and national AIDS experts that attracted the attention of the national and provincial governments and international funding agencies, which in turn facilitated and enlarged the outreach capacity and effectiveness of the HAI AIDS program in China.

One of the unique features of the Chinese AIDS medical training program was the training of the ARV therapy adhesion monitors in the AIDS villages. The function of these AIDS therapy adhesion monitors shared some similarity with the "DOT" (direct observed therapy) in the TB treatment program, except whereas monitoring for TB cases was designed to last only 3–6 months, the AIDS therapy monitoring was designed to last longer. Most of these monitors were selected from family members of the AIDS patients or their fellow villagers. After brief training about AIDS and the critical importance of the treatment adhesion in ARV therapy, the monitors were requested to witness a patient taking the medicine daily and to keep a record of the patient adhesion to the treatment. Some of the monitors were assigned as the group leaders in charge of monitoring the monitors' performance. These group leaders usually received a minimum payment for their job from the local governments.

In conclusion, building a basic health care infrastructure, educating the public about the AIDS epidemic, and training sufficient numbers of clinicians and health care workers were some of the most important prerequisite elements essential for attaining effective ARV therapy. As these elements require significant time and money to establish and maintain, and since the effectiveness of ARV therapy depends upon the condition of these elements, it is conceivable that it might take many years for the AIDS patients in resource-poor countries and regions to receive the most effective ARV therapy even when ARV drugs are readily available. Because these essential elements are a part of the general health care system for a local community, one might question if it would even be possible for some of the poorest countries or regions to provide the ARV therapy as effectively as in the rest of the world.

Therapeutic HIV Vaccines as an Adjunct to ARV Therapy

Given that the effectiveness of the ARV therapy largely depends on socioeconomic conditions such as drug availability and the existence of a basic health care system, is it possible to improve current ARV therapy in such a way that will be less dependent on a region's existing resources? The development of therapeutic HIV vaccines as an adjunct to ARV therapy (adjunct therapeutic HIV vaccine, ATHV) may provide just such a possibility.

The rationale for developing an ATHV is as follows: whereas ARV therapy can effectively inhibit the virus replication, an ATHV could stimulate cell-mediated immune (CMI) responses that kill host cells harboring the virus, which serve as the reservoirs for the appearance of drug-resistant mutant viruses. If the ATHV approach indeed works, then it is possible that ARV therapy need not be an uninterrupted lifelong therapy. This advantage of ATHV therapy may provide an additional benefit for resource-poor regions, since most ARV therapy failures in these regions result from low adhesion to the strict drug-taking schedules, which enables the appearance of drug-resistant mutant viruses. If one could enhance protective immune responses while still maintaining effective ARV therapy, such immune responses might be able to suppress the replication of drug-resistant mutant viruses even with occasional non-adhesion to the ARV therapy. In other words, ATHV may compensate for the effectiveness of ARV therapy lost due to low adhesion, thus making the first-line drug regimen last longer, and reducing the rate of the ARV treatment failure.

The following is a brief review of one of the development of ATHV products based on the scientific rationale described earlier.

In 1999, HAI researchers reported that a fragment of Anthrax lethal factor (LFn) possesses a special function that enables its entering inside an antigen-presenting cell without being degraded like other extracellular proteins [10]. In subsequent years, the HAI researchers demonstrated that after LFn was fused with an HIV virus antigen, including the Gag, Env, and Nef, respectively, as a recombinant fusion protein, the LFn–HIV fusion antigens could enter into cytosol. Once inside the cytosol of antigen-presenting cells, the HIV antigen would be processed by the classic MHC-I pathway as if the viral antigens had been produced endogenously in an infected host cell [11]. After it was shown that the LFn–HIV fusion techniques could become a new approach to make T cell vaccines that aim at eliciting antigen-specific CMI responses for protection, HAI collaborated with the Walter Reed Army Institute of the Research (WRAIR) to develop the LFn–p24C into a human vaccine candidate. This vaccine is a recombinant protein in which the LFn was fused with the p24 Gag protein from a subtype C virus isolated from southern Africa. In 2003, WRAIR successfully produced the LFn–p24C in its Forest Glen manufacturing facility in compliance with GMP. The new candidate vaccine also went through vigorous safety tests in animals in commercial testing facilities in compliance with GLP (Good Laboratory Practices) and obtained the satisfactory preclinical safety results. Finally, the candidate vaccine was tested in a phase I human clinical study in which 16 healthy American volunteers took the vaccine without showing any adverse effects of concern [12]. The satisfactory result of this human safety study led to the decision of a Boston-based US biotech company, Vaccine Technology Inc. (VTI), to license from Harvard University the worldwide exclusive rights of using this new technology platform to develop commercial products in the field of infectious diseases and in other fields as well. Soon after completing the licensing agreement with Harvard in 2004, VTI sponsored a phase I human safety trial in 30 AIDS patients in Uganda in collaboration with researchers from the California Department of Health and the Joint Clinical Research center in Kampala, Uganda.

Based on the approach described at the beginning of this section, these AIDS patients had started to receive ARV therapy effectively (virus load <400) and their immune system had not been completely destroyed by the virus (CD4 >400). While they continued their ARV therapies, their viral antigen-specific CMI responses were stimulated by receiving three consecutive intramuscular injections of the recombinant LFn–p24C over a period of 3 months. After 12 months continuous clinical observations of these patients, the researchers concluded that the LFn–p24C was safe to use as an immune therapy in AIDS patients as well as in healthy volunteers [13].

Another challenge emerged in determining how to measure the effectiveness of an ATHV. Although all the patients continued to do well in their ARV therapy, and although their CD4 cells seemed to increase after the injections, and although there

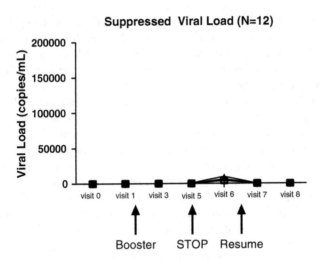

Fig. 7.2 Effect of ATHV on scheduled ARV treatment interruption [1]

was evidence that the LFn–p24C had stimulated the antigen-specific immune responses, these results could not directly confirm hopes for the ATHV concept.

If ATHV could stimulate HIV-specific cytotoxic T lymphocytes (CTL) that kill HIV-infected host cells, thus destroying the host cells that harbor the provirus integrated into the host genome, then it would be possible to stop ARV from time to time. The best possible outcome of this approach is even more staggering: if the CTL stimulated by the therapeutic HIV vaccine could destroy all infected host cells in the presence of an effective ARV drug, then it would be possible to cure AIDS.

In collaboration with the prominent Ugandan AIDS researchers in the national Joint Clinical Research Centre, and in compliance with all the international and local regulatory and ethical regulations, the researchers conducted a carefully designed study of "scheduled treatment interruptions" in the same AIDS patient volunteers who had previously received three injections of LFn–p24C as an ATHV [13]. After receiving a boost shot of the LFn–p24C, all the patients stopped taking their ARV drugs for 4 weeks, and then resumed the therapy with the same ARV regimens they used earlier. The HIV load assays were performed before, during, and after the scheduled treatment interruptions. As shown in Fig. 7.2, half of the patients had either undetectable or very low virus loads throughout the scheduled treatment interruptions. The other half had visible virus load rebounds during the scheduled treatment interruptions, but not after retaking the ARV drugs (Fig. 7.3). This was an encouraging result for the development of ATHV.

Encouraged by the initial positive clinical results, VTI's wholly owned subsidiary in China (Haikou VTI; http://www.haikouvti.com) in 2006 built a GMP manufacturing facility on the Chinese island of Hainan, aiming to apply for a product license for LFn–p24 in China. Since then, Haikou VTI has reengineered the LFn–p24C construct in order to meet SFDA's requirements. Haikou VTI has also replaced

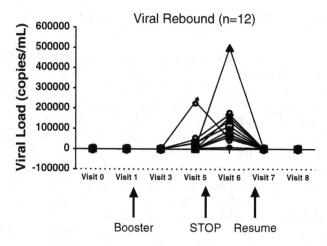

Fig. 7.3 Effect of ATHV on scheduled ARV treatment interruption [2]

the p24C of African origin with the p24 (B/C) of Chinese origin. In 2008, the Haikou VTI manufacturing facility received the GMP certificate from the provincial FDA. In 2010, Haikou VTI successfully produced three consecutive batches of the LFn–p24 (B/C) in compliance with the Chinese GMP. In 2011, after completing the pre-clinical safety studies in the SFDA certified testing facilities with satisfactory results, Haikou VTI filed the new IND application in China.

HIV Vaccines

An effective HIV vaccine will be an ideal solution to stop the spread of the AIDS pandemic; however, HIV vaccine development has not turned out to be what people expected twenty or even 10 years ago. In 1985, the then secretary of US Human and Health Services Margaret Heckler proclaimed that a vaccine would be available in 2 years. In 1997, then President Bill Clinton called for scientists to make an HIV vaccine in 10 years. Today, many scientists are debating whether it is even possible to develop an HIV vaccine. HIV is a retrovirus: once an infection occurs, its genome becomes an integrated part of a human genome. Most effective vaccines, if not all, can protect vaccine recipients from getting a disease, but cannot necessarily protect them from being infected. For the same reason, even if it is possible to develop an effective HIV vaccine, such a vaccine will not be able to eradicate the AIDS disease like the smallpox vaccine did to smallpox.

Since 1985, there have been three HIV vaccines tested in large-scale human efficacy trials. The following description provides a very brief overview of where we stand today in the field of HIV vaccine development and with the concept of HIV vaccines with ARV prophylaxis.

The First Phase III HIV Vaccine Efficacy Trial

The HIV vaccine candidate that was first tested in a phase III human efficacy trial took about 15 years from start to finish. The design of the vaccine, gp120, followed the approach of the first successful recombinant protein-based Hepatitis B vaccine, which was also the most profitable human vaccine at the time [14]. The recombinant Hepatitis B vaccine used the Hepatitis B virus's surface protein as the antigen to induce neutralizing antibodies in humans against the virus; similarly, gp120 was a recombinant protein of HIV-1 envelope protein that was shown to stimulate neutralizing antibodies in humans against HIV-1 viruses [15]. In 2005, the first human phase III trial concluded that the vaccine had no protective efficacy [16, 17]. Even before the conclusion of the human efficacy trial, most mainstream scientists already concluded that an effective HIV vaccine must stimulate CMI response in addition to neutralizing antibodies [18]. Since the recombinant gp120 could not stimulate CMI response, it alone would not be able to offer protection. The US biotech company, VaxGen, conducted the trial in Thailand and in the USA with support from the US NIH. The company abandoned its approach to use gp120 alone as an HIV vaccine soon after the conclusion of the phase III human trial.

The second phase III HIV vaccine efficacy trial tested the approach of stimulating both CMI response and neutralizing antibodies, plus a new vaccination strategy called "prime-boost." This class of vaccines usually contains at least two components, one used in the first immunization as "prime" and the other used in the subsequent immunizations of the same individuals as "boost." As this second generation of HIV vaccine candidates differed significantly from all the previous human vaccine developments and were produced with some of the most advanced biotechnologies in vaccine manufacturing, a brief description about this novel new class of vaccines may prove instructive, and is provided below.

The CMI-Based Vaccines

In order to effectively stimulate CMI responses, the HIV antigens must be expressed "in vivo," meaning inside antigen-presenting cells of a vaccine recipient. This unique feature of most CMI-based vaccines usually requires using a live viral or bacterial vector that is able to deliver a gene encoding one or more HIV antigens (as opposed to delivering the antigens themselves) into a host cell so that the HIV antigens can be expressed and synthesized as intracellular proteins. Another common approach to making a CMI-based vaccine is to use the "naked" DNA by injecting into a vaccine recipient large amounts of recombinant plasmid DNA containing HIV-1 structural genes, and letting the DNA molecules synthesize the HIV antigen inside a host cell. None of the human vaccines currently available for commercial usage has ever before been made in such a way.

The Prime-Boost Strategy

This new vaccination strategy actually was necessary for any CMI vaccine candidate using live virus vector (or live bacterial vector like salmonella), because the host immunity against the vector could interfere with subsequent immunizations using the same vector. In order to boost CMI response to the HIV antigens more effectively, the boost immunizations usually use a different type of CMI vaccine candidate, such as DNA vaccines. As aforementioned, none of the existing human vaccines require such a vaccination strategy.

The vaccine candidates tested in the second HIV vaccine phase III efficacy trial were developed by Merck, which has successfully developed many of the human vaccines in the past. In 2009, the company announced that because the rate of HIV infection in the people who received the vaccine was higher than that of the people who received only placebo, the clinic trial had to be stopped [19]. It took the company about 15 years from the beginning of the vaccine development research to the unsuccessful conclusion of the phase III trial. Like VaxGen, Merck suspended its active development program on HIV vaccines.

According to the publications after the completion of the clinical trial, one possible reason for the vaccine failure was related to the fact that some of the people who received the live virus-based vaccine in fact had preexisting immunity against the vector virus.

The third HIV vaccine phase III efficacy trial was conducted in Thailand by the US military's AIDS research program, in collaboration with the Royal Thai Army. Although the vaccine candidates tested in this trial were also designed by the same prime-boost strategy and in accordance with the principle that both CMI and neutralizing antibodies are required for protective efficacy against HIV-1, it also took into account the lessons learned from the previous two efficacy trials. First of all, the vaccine avoided using a live viral vector that may have preexisting immunity in humans. Second, it used the recombinant gp120 to specifically boost the induction of neutralizing antibodies against HIV. This vaccine trial was concluded in 2011 [20]. The result showed a protective efficacy rate of 31% for the vaccine candidates.

The full impact of this last HIV vaccine phase III efficacy trial is still unclear. To many, such a low protective efficacy should mean that the current understanding of the AIDS pathogenesis, the available technologies, and the vaccine development approaches are simply insufficient to make a successful HIV vaccine. More basic research on the virus, the human immune system, and vaccinology are needed in order to make an effective HIV vaccine, assuming an HIV vaccine is even possible to make. The more than 20 years and many US$ hundreds of millions needed to get the results of the three unsuccessful phase III efficacy trials warrant a reevaluation of current HIV vaccine development strategies. Other human vaccines usually took an average of 10 years and about US$100 million to reach the market [21]. The HIV vaccine development is obviously an exception.

When will the next HIV vaccine efficacy trial be conducted? Before answering this question, one needs to know that the HIV vaccine development is very unique in the history of the vaccine industry. Unlike all other human vaccine developments, HIV vaccine development has relied heavily on public funding for support. The US NIH has provided significant funds to all three past HIV vaccine efficacy trials, and the last vaccine trials were almost completely supported by the US government. Therefore, judging by the current pessimistic atmosphere in the public sector towards HIV vaccine development, and by the lack of active involvement from any major pharmaceutical companies to develop new vaccine candidates, it is likely that there will be no more HIV vaccine phase III efficacy trials in the near future. Consequently, it becomes more and more unlikely that there will be an effective commercial HIV vaccine available in the coming decade, or even thereafter.

In the face of a 30-year past of a continuously spreading AIDS epidemic, the thought of having no effective vaccine for the next 10 or more years is almost unbearable, especially to public health workers in developing countries. This dark picture is not, however, inevitable. The following discussion explores some possible alternative approaches to the HIV vaccine development.

ARV Prophylaxis

In 1987, the first FDA-approved anti-HIV drug AZT was recommended for use as a prophylactic treatment for hospital staff who had been accidentally exposed to the virus. Then, in 1991, it was reported that treating HIV-infected pregnant women with ARV therapy could protect unborn babies from being infected by HIV-1 before or after birth [22]. Since then, using ARV to prevent mother-to-infant transmission of HIV has become standard practice—even in some resource-poor regions (see the chapter by Dr. Zhou in this book). The success of this approach to protect unborn babies from being infected by HIV actually approved the concept of ARV prophylaxis. It has become perhaps one of the most effective public health measures in the absence of an effective HIV vaccine.

Harvard researcher Max Essex first advocated the concept of using ARV prophylaxis as a substitute HIV vaccine. In 2007, Max Essex, Bob Gallo, Bob Redfield, and Bill Haseltine proposed it again in a public meeting and published the analysis in the popular magazine "Atlantic" [23]. Since all ARV NNRT and NRT drugs act to inhibit the function of HIV-1's reverse transcriptase, thus preventing the virus from replicating in the very early stages, it is conceivable that ARV prophylaxis may even be able to prevent infections as well as disease progression, especially when using NNRT or NRT in combination with a viral entry blocker drug like T-20 [24]. If one can develop such ARV combination drugs with a long-lasting effect, ARV prophylaxis may indeed become a "substitute vaccine."

HIV Vaccines with ARV Prophylaxis

If one combines the HIV vaccines as tested in the last phase III efficacy trials together with ARV regimens that is designed to be taken periodically, will one get a more effective vaccine? In other words, can vaccine-induced neutralizing antibodies, CMI responses, and ARV act in synergy to offer effective protections? In theory, the answer is a "yes." Vaccine-induced neutralizing antibodies can prevent viruses from binding effectively with their receptors on the host cell membranes. For those viruses that escape the host protection by neutralizing antibodies, a T-20-like fusion peptide-based ARV drug can block viruses from entering into the host cells by inhibiting the fusion process between the membranes of the viruses and the host cells. For viruses that escape both neutralizing antibodies and fusion inhibitor ARV, one or more NRT and NNRT drugs can block the functions of the viral reverse transcriptase, thus preventing HIV-1 from converting its RNA genome into a DNA-based provirus that is essential for integrating the viral genome into the host genomic DNA. When viruses manage escaping all host protection listed earlier and successfully integrate into the host cell genomes, vaccine-induced CTLs can recognize and kill the infected host cells that produce new viruses. Considering the fact that the current vaccine candidates are safe to use and can stimulate neutralizing antibodies and CTLs, and that NRT/NNRT/T-20 ARV regimens have been used safely and effectively, testing such a hypothetical HIV vaccine with ARV prophylaxis should be feasible.

There may be various ways to use the proposed HIV vaccines with ARV prophylaxis by applying the ARV components periodically according to high-risk factors associated with particular communities who receive the vaccine.

Summary

As should by now be evident, there is not a simple answer to the question asked at the beginning of this chapter. Any answer will have to depend on several unknown factors, including the global supplies of generic ARV drugs in the coming years, the level of the international and domestic funding to provide ARV drugs and help to build the necessary public health infrastructures, and the successful product developments of ATHV and HIV vaccines. Figure 7.4 was used in the discussions during the HAI's AIDS medical training courses and workshops in China to illustrate the impact and relationship between these factors. This figure was formulated as a socioeconomic balance between the global supply of, and demand for, ARV therapy.

The Availability of ARV Drugs May Not Improve Significantly in the Next 10 Years

According to the UNAIDS' latest report, there were 33.3 million people living with HIV/AIDS worldwide who either needed ARV therapy now or in the near future. In 2009, about 5.25 million AIDS patients received ARV therapy [25]. Approximately 90% of these patients lived in low- and middle-income countries and relied on public funding for their ARV drug supplies and treatment monitoring and counseling.

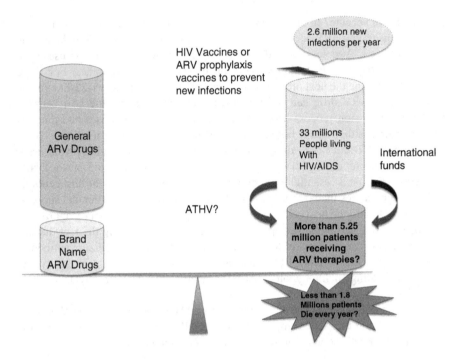

Fig. 7.4 Global demand and supply of ARV therapy

Thus far, the biggest resource for public funding came from the US Presidential Emergency Program for AIDS Research (PEPFAR), which provided US$ six billion in 2009 alone to support the ARV therapy in developing countries, and especially in Africa [26].

Since its inception in 2002, PEPFAR has provided more than US$32 billion to support ARV therapies in developing countries where AIDS therapy was badly needed but unavailable without significant outside financial help. In many ways, PEPFAR has become the most significant driving force in making effective ARV therapy available to more AIDS patients in the resource-poor countries or regions. In order to make ARV therapy available to more AIDS patients who need it, the best hope seems to rely on the US government to expand the current PEPFAR or to expand, together with other industrial nations, international funding agencies such as the Global Funds.

Realistically, however, there are growing concerns about how long PEPFAR can last, and whether the program can even maintain at the current level of the funding. As effective ARV therapies should be lifelong therapies, the consequences of interrupting the therapies because of discontinuous financial support would be nothing but disastrous. Judging by the performance of the global economy in the past few years, and by the heated US domestic political debates about the current US federal deficit, one cannot help worrying about the future of programs such as PEPFAR and

Global Funds. It may actually take much longer to make effective ARV therapies to most AIDS patients in the world than any of us had anticipated before the 2008 global financial crisis.

Without international funding to resource-poor countries and regions, the high cost of the ARV drugs is simply unattainable for the majority of AIDS patients in the world. In 2009, the weighted cost of the first-line regimen for an AIDS patient in low- and middle-incomes was about $141 per year, and $1378 per year for the second-line regimen.

If resource-poor countries cannot count on international funding to finance the ARV therapy in their own countries, they will have to search for an alternative solution. Given the weighted costs for ARV treatment listed earlier, the potential global market for the first-line regimen will be about US$ 4,695 million and $15,158 million for the second-line regimen, assuming 1/3 of the AIDS patients receiving the first line ARV treatment will require a second-line regimen. In the coming decade, when the patent protections for most of the current brand name ARV drugs will gradually expire, one of the most effective and reliable ways to improve access to ARV drugs is for developing countries to build their own drug manufacturers. In fact, some countries, such as India, South Africa, Brazil, Thailand, and China, have already had success in this endeavor. Others, such as Uganda, Tanzania, Zambia, Ghana, and Zimbabwe, have also made significant progress towards this goal. It is possible that after 2020, these developing countries could become self-sufficient in their domestic need for ARV drugs, and the resource-poor countries could purchase ARV drugs from the most cost-effective international suppliers.

Unfortunately, the current situation will become worse before it gets better. There were 2.6 million new HIV infections and 1.8 million deaths caused by AIDS in 2009 [25]. If this trend continues, both the number of the people who need ARV therapy and the number of AIDS patients who need continuous support for their ARV therapy will increase at a faster rate, thus further outpacing new ARV therapy and HIV vaccine developments.

The Essential Public Health Infrastructures in Resource-Poor Countries May Not Improve Significantly in the Next 10 Years

As discussed in previous sections, an effective ARV therapy requires basic health care infrastructure such as medical counseling and clinical monitoring, as well as lifelong ARV drug supplies. Such basic health care infrastructures simply do not exist in resource-poor countries and regions, and building such infrastructure is far beyond the financial capacities of the local governments without outside help. According to the PEPFAR expenditures in the past several years, these international aid programs need to double or quadruple in size within the next few years in order to meet the growing global demands for effective ARV therapies. Given the current state of funding programs and public support, this is unlikely to happen.

ATHV Can Make the Global ARV Therapy Possible

The most difficult part of an effective ARV therapy is its requirement of lifelong treatment. If an ATHV described in the previous sections can destroy the remaining host cells that harbor the virus, thus eliminating the potential reservoir in which the virus can replicate, then it can fundamentally change the prospects for future ARV therapy. In other words, if AIDS can be cured, and not require lifelong medical treatment, then making the therapy available to most AIDS patients in the world can become feasible in the foreseeable future.

New HIV Infections Have to Be Reduced Significantly Before most AIDS Patients in the World Can Receive Effective ARV Therapies

Without a cure for AIDS, effective ARV therapies require more and more AIDS patients to depend on financial support to survive, thus creating a snowball effect on the growing demand for public health resources to the point where therapy becomes unaffordable. Without an effective HIV vaccine candidate on the horizon, an HIV vaccine with ARV prophylaxis may be the most effective method to prevent new HIV infections.

In conclusion, if the current international financial support can be increased very significantly, then it is possible for most AIDS patients in the world to receive effective ARV therapy in the next 10 years. If AIDS can be cured by ARV therapy with a therapeutic HIV vaccine, then it is also possible to treat most AIDS patients in the world. The global public health programs on TB treatment and prevention offer just such precedents. Finally, an effective HIV vaccine, with or without ARV prophylaxis, offers the best solution to prevent future generations of public health workers from having to face the challenges of AIDS forever.

References

1. Carpenter CC, Fischl MA, Hammer SM, Hirsch MS, Jacobsen DM, Katzenstein DA, Montaner JS, Richman DD, Saag MS, Schooley RT, Thompson MA, Vella S, Yeni PG, Volberding PA (1997) Antiretroviral therapy for HIV infection in 1997: Updated recommendations of the International AIDS Society-USA panel. JAMA 277:1962–1969
2. Cascade Collaboration (2003) Determinants of survival following HIV-1 seroconversion after the introduction of HAART. Lancet 362:1267–1274
3. Cai Deshan (2010) 21 antiretroviral drugs approved by SFDA. Chinese Medicine Economic News 2010.12.10 (http://health.sohu.com/20101210/n278226750.shtml)
4. Lu Y, Essex M (eds) (2006) AIDS in Asia. Springer, New York
5. Essex M, Mboop S, Kanki P, Marlink R, Tlou S (eds) (2002) AIDS in Africa. Kluwer, New York
6. Alice Park (2005) AIDS whistle-blower. Time Magazine 2005, Oct 31. (http://www.time.com/time/magazine/article/0,9171,1124297,00.html)
7. Gui X (2008) In: Lu Y, Essex M (eds) Emerging Infections in Asia. Springer, New York

8. UNAIDS (2002) HIV/AIDS: China's titanic peril. June 2002
9. Bussmann C, Ndwapi N, Gaolathe T, Bussmann H, Wester CW, Ncube P et al (2004) Supporting national ART scale-up in Botswana through standardized, multi-phased training (http://ftguonline.org/ftgu-232/index.php/ftgu/article/view/1946/3888). Also see: The Botswana Ministry of Health and KITSO Planning Committee: KITSO Expansion Plan (2004) The full KITSO Medical Training manual can be downloaded from http://www.hiv.gov.bw/uploads/KITSO%20Plan%20FINAL.pdf
10. Kushner N, Zhang D, Touzjian N, Essex M, Lieberman J, Lu Y (2003) A fragment of anthrax lethal factor delivers proteins to the cytosol without requiring protective antigen. Proc Natl Acad Sci USA 100:6652–6657
11. Cao H, Agrawal D, Kushner N, Touzjian N, Essex M, Lu Y (2002) Delivery of exogenous protein antigens to major histocompatibility complex class I pathway in cytosol. J Infect Dis 185:244–251
12. WRAIR: RV 151: A phase I study of safety and immunogenicity of the WRAIR HIV-1 vaccine LFn-p24 administered by the intramuscular (IM) route in healthy adults. WRAIR #984, HSRRB Log # A-11905 (http://apps.who.int/trialsearch/trial.aspx?trialid=NCT00412477)
13. Kityo C, Bousheri S, Akao J, Ssali F, Byaruhanga R, Ssewanyana I et al (2011) Therapeutic immunization in HIV infected Ugandans receiving stable antiretroviral treatment: a phase I safety study. Vaccine 29(8):1617–1623
14. Murray K (1989) Success stories...pioneering development of Hepatitis B vaccine. Edinburgh Research and Innovation (http://www.research-innovation.ed.ac.uk/success/hepatitisB.asp)
15. Shao Y, Lu Y (1999) Biodiversity and bioseparation of HIV-1 envelope glycoproteins. Crit Rev Oncog 10:1–16
16. Flynn NM, Forthal DN, Harro CD, Judson FN, Mayer KH, Para MF (2005) Placebo-controlled phase 3 trial of a recombinant 760 glycoprotein 120 vaccine to prevent HIV-1 infection. J Infect Dis 191:654–665
17. Pitisuttithum P, Gilbert P, Gurwith M, Heyward W, Martin M, van Griensven F, Hu D, Tappero JW, Choopanya K (2006) Randomized, double-blind, placebo- 762 controlled efficacy trial of a bivalent recombinant glycoprotein 120 HIV-1 vaccine among 763 injection drug users in Bangkok, Thailand. J Infect Dis 194:1661–1671
18. Korber BT, Letvin NL, Haynes BF (2009) T-cell vaccine strategies for human immunodeficiency virus, the virus with a thousand faces. J Virol 83:8300–8314
19. Buchbinder S, Mehrotra D, Duerr A, Fitzgerald D, Mogg R, Li D et al (2008) Efficacy assessment of a cell-mediated immunity HIV-1 vaccine (the Step Study): a double-blind, randomised, placebo-controlled, test-of-concept trial. Lancet 373:1881–1893
20. Rerks-Ngarm S, Pitisuttithum P, Nitayaphan S, Kaewkungwal J, Chiu J, Paris R, Premsri N, Namwat C, de Souza M, Adams E, Benenson M, Gurunathan S, Tartaglia J, McNeil JG, Francis DP, Stablein D, Birx DL, Chunsuttiwat S, Khamboonruang C, Thongcharoen P, Robb ML, Michael NL, Kunasol P, Kim JH (2009) 770 Vaccination with ALVAC and AIDSVAX to prevent HIV-1 infection in Thailand. New Engl J 771 Med 361:2212–2220
21. Somers J, Webre P (2008) US policy regarding pandemic-influenza vaccines, Chap 2. Developing new vaccines Box 2-1; vaccine development: typical time and cost (http://www.cbo.gov/ftpdocs/95xx/doc9573/Chapter2.6.1.shtml#1093315)
22. Siegfried N, van der Merwe L, Brocklehurst P, Sint TT (2011) Antiretrovirals for reducing the risk of mother-to-child transmission of HIV infection. Cochrane Database Syst Rev
23. The Atlantic Magazine (2009) An early end to the HIV/AIDS pandemic? 25 Feb 2009
24. Raffi F (2004) Clinical efficacy and tolerance of enfuvirtide (Fuzeon), new antiretroviral inhibitors of intracellular penetration of human immunodeficiency virus (HIV) type 1. Medecine et Maladies Infectieuses 34(1):8–17
25. United Nations Program on HIV/AIDS. http://www.unaids.org
26. The United States President's emergency plan for AIDS relief. http://www.pepfar.gov

Index